LEADING A HOSPITAL TURNAROUND
A PRACTICAL GUIDE

LEADING A HOSPITAL TURNAROUND
A PRACTICAL GUIDE

Anthony K. Jones

ACHE Management Series

Your board, staff, or clients may also benefit from this book's insight. For more information on quantity discounts, contact the Health Administration Press Marketing Manager at (312) 424–9470.

This publication is intended to provide accurate and authoritative information in regard to the subject matter covered. It is sold, or otherwise provided, with the understanding that the publisher is not engaged in rendering professional services. If professional advice or other expert assistance is required, the services of a competent professional should be sought.

The statements and opinions contained in this book are strictly those of the author and do not represent the official positions of the American College of Healthcare Executives or the Foundation of the American College of Healthcare Executives.

17   16   15   14   13   5   4   3   2   1

Library of Congress Cataloging-in-Publication Data
Jones, Anthony K.
 Leading a hospital turnaround : a practical guide / authored by Anthony K. Jones.
  pages cm
 ISBN 978-1-56793-591-2 (alk. paper)
 1. Hospitals--Business management. 2. Health facilities--Finance. 3. Strategic planning.
4. Organizational change. 5. Leadership. I. Title.
 RA971.3.J66 2014
 362.11068--dc23
                          2013006348

The paper used in this publication meets the minimum requirements of American National Standard for Information Sciences—Permanence of Paper for Printed Library Materials, ANSI Z39.48-1984. ∞ ™

Acquisitions editor: Carrie McDonald; Project manager: Amy Carlton; Cover designer: Marisa Jackson; Layout: Virginia Byrne

Found an error or a typo? We want to know! Please e-mail it to hap1@ache.org, and put "Book Error" in the subject line.

For photocopying and copyright information, please contact Copyright Clearance Center at www.copyright.com or at (978) 750–8400.

Health Administration Press
A division of the Foundation of the American
  College of Healthcare Executives
One North Franklin Street, Suite 1700
Chicago, IL 60606–3529
(312) 424–2800

To my family,
Sheila T. Gregory, Courtney G. Jones, and Anthony K. Jones II.
Your patience, understanding, and encouragement in the writing of
this book will be forever appreciated.

and

to my former colleagues,
Loren Chandler, Michael Davenport, Denise Dillard,
Lynda Goldman, Ian McFadden, Shelly Major, and Beth Sullivan.
Thank you for providing me with the inspiration to write this book.

Contents

Preface

I GOT THE IDEA for writing this book after coleading the financial turnaround of a multihospital system. Though I have been involved in numerous difficult turnarounds, I found this one by far the most difficult. It was also the most successful. Being able to lift an organization's performance well beyond your expectations, as well as those of others, can have a lasting effect on what you think is possible.

Having served as CEO and COO in multiple hospitals and hospital systems, I wrote this book from a CEO's perspective. *Leading a Hospital Turnaround: A Practical Guide* is intended to be an honest conversation about the challenges CEOs may face when they find themselves in a financial turnaround. That means that sometimes the advice in this book will not be flattering, but it will be on point. Several good books have been written on turnarounds. However, none has reached the technical specificity and emotional depth this book offers.

If you do not know where to start in a turnaround, this book is a great place to begin. It walks through the entire turnaround process from beginning to end with practical advice based on my years of experience. It equips you with the methods and tools necessary to perform the initial diagnostic process on your organization. Detailed recommendations help you structure your communications process. Engagement strategies are suggested for working with your key stakeholders. Turnaround team member roles and responsibilities are defined in a way that leaves little doubt about who should be doing what.

In turnarounds, the things not said can have just as chilling an effect on relationships as those that are said. This book goes into great detail about how to handle these situations. Unlike other books on the subject, this book asks the reader to go through a personal self-examination process as she prepares to lead a turnaround. It advises the reader to set aside his ego for a short time and recognize the pivotal leadership tipping points that could await him.

This book is not about long-term strategies—it is about boots-on-the-ground tactics that can be accomplished immediately. At the end of each chapter you will find a checklist of critical success factors (CSFs), concrete steps that illustrate the concepts discussed in the chapter. The CSFs provide a to-do list for executives and turnaround teams to implement during a turnaround. Each chapter's CSFs build on those of the previous chapters. The CSFs can be combined and used as quick reference guide. They can be structured into a discussion document for your team and key stakeholders. The CSFs eliminate some of the complexity that all too frequently surrounds a turnaround process.

This book is intended to be a how-to book, companion, and survival guide all in one, and its step-by-step format should make for an easy read. There is no cookie-cutter approach to financial turnarounds. But these proven methods can have a lasting positive effect on your career.

—Anthony K. Jones

CHAPTER 1

Predicting a Crisis: Early Warning Signs

THE LEAD-UP

Hospital turnarounds traditionally have been viewed as institutions gradually lapsing into financial decline. Eventually, the decline takes an aggregate financial toll on the organization and reaches a trigger point. This situation still happens regularly.

But today, environments can change rapidly. Even historically well-run institutions' financial fortunes can go sour because of changes and shifts in the market. Any institution can be subject to financial decline if its leadership is not vigilant. However, few healthcare institutions drift into financial distress without having telegraphed some early warning signs.

Other than in hospitals struggling visibly with their bottom lines, identifying circumstances where a hospital is trending toward serious financial distress is not easy, but it is possible. Sometimes the signs are unmistakable. An example of distress could be the leadership's concern about the organization's ability to pay its bills. Another sign might be a decision to cut back on the level and type of services offered to the community. More common are the institutions in the middle of the road experiencing fluctuating cash flow streams simply from earning less money than they are spending.

For the vast majority of hospitals, discovering signs of distress requires a thorough vetting of many factors both financial and nonfinancial. A primary objective of the CEO and senior leadership should be to make a distinction between what is a short-term hiccup—one or two quarters of losses in a fiscal year, but a positive financial outlook beyond that point—and what is a more deep-seated downturn—such as losses for more than two quarters with a continued negative financial outlook. Another example is the organization that moves back and forth between being profitable and losing money over a 12-month period. This yo-yo effect signals instability in the management system and should be treated as one potentially requiring a turnaround.

Leaders should make every effort to get a handle on the situation quickly. With each passing day, the situation is less likely to get better on its own.

Performance Analytics

When answers are needed right away, hospital leadership should gather and use performance analytics. Three basic methods exist for gathering performance analytics and getting a quick read on the organization's financial performance: the acid test, the quick test, and the comprehensive test, as shown in Exhibit 1.1. All three tests help you gather and analyze information rapidly. However, each test has a specific formula and purpose. Selecting which test to use depends on how much detail the leadership wants to delve into and how fast the information is needed.

All three tests can be developed by the chief financial officer (CFO) without spending much time or energy. Each test combines a section of key performance indicators into a snapshot of how the organization is doing. Most of information and data should already be available internally. In addition, other benchmarking data can be obtained free of charge from public agencies. Benchmarking information can also be purchased from

Exhibit 1.1: Checklist for Rapid Assessments of Hospital Financial Health

Performance Indicators (within range?)	Acid Test	Quick Test	Comprehensive Test	Purpose of Measurement
Operating margin (EBITDA) (declining or negative)	✓	✓	✓	Ability to pay short-term bills
Days cash on hand (below industry standards)	✓	✓	✓	Ability to pay short-term bills
Debt service coverage (declining ability to pay)	✓	✓	✓	Ability to pay short-term bills
Average days in accounts receivable (above industry standards)		✓	✓	Cash flow management
Average days in accounts payable (above industry standards)		✓	✓	Cash flow management
Admissions trend (up/down)		✓	✓	Physician loyalty
Emergency room volume (up/down)		✓	✓	Physician loyalty
Surgical volume (up/down)		✓	✓	Physician loyalty
Labor cost (as a percent of net revenues)			✓	Cost management
Supply and purchased services cost (as a % of net revenues)			✓	Cost management
Productivity (FTEs/adjusted occupied bed)			✓	Operational efficiency
Market share trend (up/down)			✓	Competitive position

proprietary companies. The number of vendors selling health and hospital benchmarking data has exploded in the past decade.

The Acid Test

The acid test is the quickest to perform. It zooms in on the profitability and answers the question, "Do we have enough money coming in to pay our short-term bills, including meeting payroll?"

The formula for the acid test contains indicators for operating margin, days cash on hand, and debt service coverage. Each of these indicators is a standalone performance indicator that can have a significant impact on paying short-term bills. The number of days cash on hand will be the most critical indicator of short-term financial health.

The Quick Test

The quick test uses the acid test results as a baseline and then builds cash flow and physician loyalty measures on top of it. In the quick test, you want to know if you are properly balancing cash coming in with cash going out. Leadership's ability to manage this balance is critical to a successful turnaround. The goal in cash flow management is to pull in as much cash as possible from generated business and other sources, such as the sale of noncore assets. On the other side of the ledger, you have accounts payable, where your goal will be to pace your payment process (cash outflow) to vendors to reflect the money you are bringing in (cash inflows).

The quick test will also help you determine if the level of business flowing through the organization is stable enough to generate the level of financial strength necessary to keep the organization on track and moving forward. Here, examining volume statistics comes into play. One pointed question to answer is how well your organization is doing with admissions, surgical cases, and emergency department visits. Look for swings and patterns in these areas, which could dramatically affect organizational revenues. Within each service line, start the process by reviewing the admitting patterns of major admitters. Do any patterns here suggest a significant change in loyalty to the organization?

The Comprehensive Test

The comprehensive test uses the results of the acid and quick tests as a baseline and integrates discussions about cost management, operational efficiency, and the organization's competitive position in the market. Labor, supply, and purchased services expenses will constitute between 80 and 90 percent of total operating expenses. Getting a handle on where you stand on these important indicators is a must. While many hospital and organizational productivity indicators exist, one of the more commonly used indicators for comparative purposes measures full-time equivalent employees (FTEs) and adjusted occupied beds. This number can provide an immediate snapshot of how the organization is performing in personnel staffing.

Analyzing Leading and Lagging Indicators

One of the more common mistakes hospital leaders make when delving into the diagnostic aspects of a turnaround is to focus solely on lagging indicators and not pay attention to the leading indicators. The terms *leading* and *lagging indicators* describe the qualitative and quantitative performance of an organization within a financial context. Leading indicators precede the visibility of lagging indicators and the deterioration process. Leading indicators are the causes of financial distress, while lagging indicators are the symptoms. Examples of some leading and lagging indicators can be found in Exhibit 1.2.

Lagging indicators include routinely reported statistics and ratios found in most institutions' financial statements. These indicators must be reviewed, but experience suggests going further upstream to look at situations, events, and decisions that may be the root causes of performance deficits. The lagging indicators tell you where you are but not how you got there. The "how" question can be answered by looking at the leading indicators. Leading indicators are the bellwether for an organization in financial distress—they can predict what is to come in the lagging indicators, but they often go ignored or unnoticed until the financial deterioration has reached a threatening or critical stage. Once the lagging indicators are on the books, you may already be in damage-control mode. Do not take leading indicators for granted.

Exhibit 1.2: Leading and Lagging Performance Indicators

Leading indicators (causes)	Volume	Increasing, decreasing, or neutral? Especially for inpatient admissions, OR cases, ED visits, outpatient visits.
	Market share	Increasing, decreasing, or neutral? Overall rank and service line rank in the competitive market?
	Physician loyalty	Profile each physician. Are their admissions increasing, decreasing, or neutral?
	Patient satisfaction	Rising, falling, or neutral? How do patients answer the question "Would you recommend this hospital?"
	Quality and clinical outcomes	Performance on quality core measures and patient safety? Performance compared to regulatory requirements and benchmarked best practices?
	Image and reputation	Improving or declining? Internally and externally?
	Management and employee turnover	Benchmarking against local competitors? Against industry standards? Trending (monthly and annually)?
	Information and data	Is available, accurate, credible, and used in the decision-making process?
	Reimbursement and payer mix	Is there erosion? Are there collection issues?
Lagging indicators (symptoms)	Operating margins	Increasing, decreasing, or neutral? Benchmarking against industry standards? Trending (monthly and annually)?
	Days in accounts receivable	Increasing, decreasing, or neutral? Benchmarking against industry standards? Trending (monthly and annually)?
	Days in accounts payables	Increasing, decreasing, or neutral? Benchmarking against industry standards? Trending (monthly and annually)?
	Days cash on hand	Increasing, decreasing, or neutral? Benchmarking against industry standards? Trending (monthly and annually)?
	Liquidity (beyond days cash on hand)	The availability of short-term assets for conversion, if needed?
	Debt service ratio	Is net income sufficient to cover annual debt service?

(continued)

Exhibit 1.2: Leading and Lagging Performance Indicators (continued)

	Bond rating	Investment grade? Increasing or declining?
	Capital investments in core business and infrastructure	Increasing, decreasing, or neutral? Higher than average age of physical plant? Deferment of mission-critical projects? Deferment of life safety projects? Higher than average age physical plant?
	Pension liability and payroll taxes	Increasing liabilities? Delayed payments?

If you view and address them appropriately, you have time to fix the issues and have a significant impact on the performance of the lagging indicators. Locating and analyzing leading indicators can help enhance a leadership team's decision-making process and accelerate the necessary course corrections.

To ensure effective financial performance, management should develop a process in which the indicators are normally part of the management reporting and oversight process, such as at weekly or biweekly executive team meetings and monthly board of directors and medical staff meetings. One of the better ways to achieve this oversight is to place the indicators in an organization's balanced scorecard performance measurement system (see Chapter 5).

COMMON CAUSES OF FINANCIAL DISTRESS

As you embark on the diagnostic journey of a turnaround, one of the first issues to address is what happened, and more important, how it happened. If your first response is that our industry is unique, stop talking! You are about to stroll down the road of excuses, and you should be on the road to finding solutions. Of course healthcare—hospitals in particular—is unique. But so are banking, airlines, automotive, and so on. The real question is, within this field, why do some organizations succeed and others fail?

The American Hospital Association (AHA) produces an annual financial trend publication on how well hospitals in all sectors are performing in aggregate with respect to operating margins. In the 2013 *Trendwatch Chartbook*, the AHA reported on hospital industry performance from 1995 to 2011. The percentage of hospitals reporting negative operating margins ranged from approximately 28 percent in 2011 to 42 percent in 2000. A regression line drawn through this chart shows approximately 30 percent of hospitals are experiencing annual operating losses.

The flip side is that about 70 percent of the hospitals had positive operating margins.

How can an industry have a consistently high level of losses that is so common that losses appear to be structurally woven into the management practices and reporting process? The usual suspects for operating losses are

- reimbursement,
- mission,
- location,
- age of facilities,
- market saturation,
- access to capital,
- recruitment, and
- culture.

Some of the structural questions can be answered in how the industry operates. Healthcare is highly competitive, but it is also a "me too" industry. This approach can be particularly true of hospitals. Being left behind is not an option, so expediency has crept into some leaders' decision-making processes. In other words, leaders veer off the road of sound decision making and start to substitute copycat strategies, copycat investments, and copycat decisions, all for the sake of expediency. A follow-

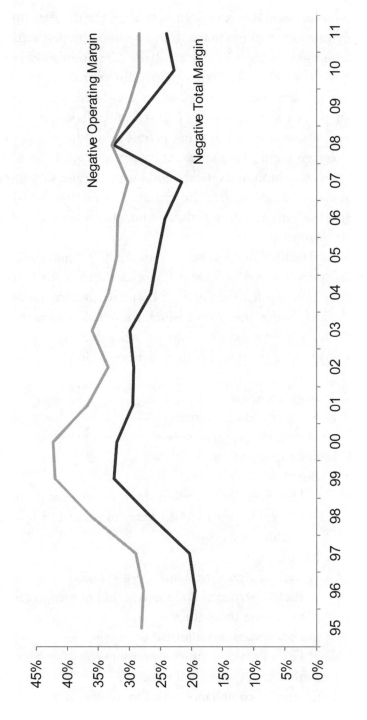

Exhibit 1.3: Percentage of Hospitals with Negative Total and Operating Margins, 1995–2011

Source: Reprinted from *Trendwatch Chartbook* by permission, copyright 2013, American Hospital Association.

the-leader mentality can lead you over a cliff. Attempting to duplicate what others have done, without proper vetting and forethought, likely will not yield the same outcomes. Deploying the same or similar strategy in a different environment with different circumstances can lead to a different result. A classic example is the acquisition of physician practices by hospitals. Many hospitals were acquiring practices but did not know how to manage them. Another example is the acquisition of health plans. Losses mounted quickly, and hospital leadership soon realized they did not possess the expertise to manage health plans. Instead of jumping on trends, do your due diligence and follow your own path.

The Health Care Advisory Board (2000) conducted a study of hospital and health system financial turnarounds. The study methodically peeled the onion of hospitals' performance layer by layer, identifying numerous common mistakes leaders made that pushed their organizations into financial decline. The Advisory Board grouped the mistakes into four categories:

1. Strategic missteps
   a. Mergers and acquisitions
   b. Diversifying beyond the core business
2. Leadership shortfalls
   a. Board of directors
      – Dissention or confusion about priorities and process
      – Critical information necessary to make decisions not reaching the board
   b. Management
      – Lack of clear direction for organization
      – Lack of technical and managerial knowledge necessary to execute successfully
      – Lots of data, no information
      – Fear of making difficult decisions
3. Organizational culture and structure
   a. Culture of compliance with the status quo

    b. Culture where relationships take precedence over sound business practices

    c. Organizational structure that is bloated and bureaucratic

4. Performance management and track record

    a. Downward trend in key performance indicators

    b. Unrealistic performance targets given the environment

    c. Expectations and performance set too low

    d. Cumulative track record of not achieving agreed-on targets

These same mistakes continue today. Strategic missteps have a profoundly negative impact on the well-being of an organization. Nowhere is this impact seen more clearly than on the balance sheets of financially distressed organizations. Strategic decisions can require large sums of capital. If an executed strategy does not pay off, it can become a financial drain in the form of declining liquidity, declining net worth, and rising debt. All of these problems surface on the balance sheet long before you see them on an income statement. The Advisory Board (2000) discovered two main contributors to strategic missteps—mergers and acquisitions, and diversification beyond an organization's core business. For example, acquiring competing hospitals that have historically had losing bottom lines or merging with another struggling hospital to reduce competition or seek economies of scale, which rarely materialize. From a diversification standpoint, some organizations make conscious decisions to purchase and manage physician practices or to own and operate health plans. Many of these strategies are recycled through the industry. But financially successful organizations rarely lose sight of their core business: managing the hospital.

Second, leadership shortfalls were detected at multiple levels within financially distressed organizations, on the board of directors and within the senior management ranks. These leadership shortfalls can be painfully obvious. Figuring out this part of the diagnostic process does not take long. Review financial statements and strategic plans, assess productivity, review board minutes, and interview key stakeholders. This information should give you a quick sense of whether the organization has leadership issues. There is no substitute for effective leadership; without it, the organization will suffer.

The third category, organizational culture, is frequently overlooked in the turnaround process because it is considered a soft area (intangible) and cannot be turned around on a dime. Also, people get downright offended if you tell them there may be a problem with their system of beliefs and practices. Organizations in turnaround tend to have affection for the status quo. In financially distressed institutions, relationships can trump sound business practices. To improve the organization's performance, leadership has to sidestep the old saying that "you have to go along to get along." To create a culture of accountability, the mold may have to be broken and the culture reshaped.

Setting and monitoring performance is the fourth and final category. Financially distressed institutions often lack a comprehensive, documented, and enforced performance management system that serves as a compass for accountability. Some of the more basic questions to ask when developing a sound performance management system include the following:

- What is the team or organization trying to accomplish?
- Who is trying to accomplish it?
- When will it be accomplished?
- Are the performance expectations measurable and set in advance?
- How is accountability handled if targets are not met?

One example of performance measurements affecting a turnaround would be having a goal of moving the hospital's cost per adjusted admission from the twenty-fifth percentile up to the seventy-fifth percentile in your peer group. Another example would be moving the FTEs/adjusted occupied bed productivity performance indicator from the twenty-fifth percentile to the seventy-fifth percentile in your peer group.

On a final note, decision making deserves a deeper discussion even though it has been mentioned before. Decision making is at the nexus of each of the four common mistakes. If an organization finds itself in a financial hole, its leaders should take the time to honestly reflect on their decisions and the decision-making process.

- Did specific thought processes or patterns lead up to the decisions that made for good judgment or not-so-good judgment?
- How was information gathered and vetted?
- Was critical information overlooked or unavailable?
- Did key individuals participate (or not participate) in the decisions?
- Were checks and balances in place?
- Were previous mistakes used as teachable moments for the current processes?
- How were the final decisions made?
- Who made the final decisions?
- What could have been done differently to have a better outcome?

BEWARE OF LEADERSHIP TIPPING POINTS

Malcolm Gladwell (2002) defines a tipping point as the "moment of critical mass, the threshold, the boiling point." Others have described a tipping point as a point at which a slow, reversible change becomes irreversible, often with dramatic consequences.

Hospital turnarounds have recognizable tipping points, especially for leaders. Triggering these tipping points can have dire consequences on you as the leader of a turnaround. Your ability to recover and seriously lead a turnaround will be difficult if people question your leadership on the basis of a lapse in judgment or other negative event. Some tipping points have fatal consequences, others are critical and lead to being fatal, and others can start out as serious and become critical if they are not addressed. Examples of serious, critical, and fatal leadership tipping points are listed in Exhibit 1.4.

Many times the tipping points and the actions leading up to them can become intertwined, creating a domino effect when one critical mass point or change can cause the deterioration of another situation. This can accelerate a downward spiral. Stay mindful of the interconnectedness of your decisions and the events that may result. For example, a no-confidence vote by the medical staff could trigger a loss of board support. If the image and reputation of the organization falls below expectations, it can trigger a lack of confidence in the leadership. A sentinel event could cause the image and reputation of the organization to fall below expectations. A no-confidence vote by the medical staff could trigger a precipitous decline in volume. A downward change in credit worthiness could restrict access to capital and cause concerns about financial viability.

Exhibit 1.4: Categories of Leadership Tipping Points

	Occurrences
Serious	• Performance falls below expectations of board or corporate leadership • A major failed decision • A sentinel event (quality or nonquality) • Bond ratings declining below investment grade
Critical	• Performance below expectation of board and corporate leadership which has not been corrected after mutual agreement to do. • No plan developed for course correction of organization • Change in political direction of internal or external supporters • Being seen as lacking competence for the job • Volume falling off the cliff • Image and reputation of the organization falling below expectations
Fatal	• Loss of confidence by the board • Loss of support from the board • A no-confidence vote by the medical staff • Continued financial losses with or without a financial turnaround plan

---

The best way to handle these types of tipping points is to be aware of them, and develop and execute your turnaround plan in a manner that does not allow reversible situations and events to become irreversible. For example:

- Have an open and direct line of communication with the board of directors and board chair. Ensure the turnaround plan has been presented and approved by the board. Schedule routine meetings for update and progress.
- Ensure the turnaround plan has been discussed in broad terms with medical staff leadership. You may not be able to get full agreement on a specific plan because of the diversity of opinions, but you should be able to gain support for a specific direction for the organization. Keep the medical staff engaged in the process through routine updates and progress reports.
- Work to ensure no surprises. If difficult messages need to be delivered or decisions made, deliver the messages and acknowledge the difficult decisions required.
- Vet major decisions prior to implementation. Decisions should not be made in a vacuum or in isolation.
- Do not underestimate the element of time. If an organization is in the red, remaining there is detrimental to leadership and the organization. Move through the process with a calm and rapid sense of purpose.
- Be mindful of an organization's image and reputation. Any decisions affecting this area should be discussed with the board and other organizational leadership.

Critical Success Factors Checklist		
CSF 1.1	Distinguish between a short-term financial hiccup and a more deep-seated financial downturn.	☐
CSF 1.2	Get a quick read on your financial situation— perform an acid test or quick test to gauge the organization's financial health.	☐
CSF 1.3	Identify both leading and lagging performance indicators. Cash flow and days cash on hand should be the first measures assessed.	☐
CSF 1.4	As early as possible, diagnose causes of organizational financial distress and any missteps. Separate symptoms from causes. (Fixing symptoms does not solve the problems.)	☐
CSF 1.5	Assess whether the organization's decision-making process is sound. Is it effective?	☐
CSF 1.6	Avoid leadership tipping points.	☐
CSF 1.7	Chart the potential domino effects of the tipping points and the actions that lead up to them. Gauge your proximity.	☐

CHAPTER 2

Facing the Facts:
Leadership Front and Center

THE HIGHER YOU rise in an organization, the more difficult it can be to admit your mistakes. Financial malaise can occur if senior leaders allow their pride to get in the way of solving problems.

OWN UP TO THE SITUATION

When a hospital CEO and her team are given the mantle of leadership for an organization, they are explicitly expected to perform at the highest level and carry out their duties in good conscience. But what happens when this does not occur?

Hospital CEOs and their leadership teams are the highest ranking individuals in the institution, other than the board of directors. At this level, the hubris of healthy egos can be omnipresent. The larger the ego, the more difficult it can be to face the facts and admit when something goes wrong on your watch.

Counterproductive egotistical thinking can saturate the thought process, including:

- If I admit there is a problem, what will this say about my leadership skills?

- How will I ever be able to answer questions about how we got here?
- Certainly I can't tell them we had other priorities that required my attention and I took my eye off the ball!

Leaders who find themselves in a turnaround should first be sure not to trip over their egos. Admitting mistakes is the first step toward correcting the problems. As early as possible, get over yourself and pivot in the direction of dealing with the serious situation at hand. Then start mapping out plans to get the organization back on track.

RESOLVING CAUSES OF MANAGEMENT INACTION

What happened? CEOs and senior leadership should be prepared to answer this question ad nauseam. While the ship was drifting off course, what were you doing? The frightening answer in many distressed situations may sound a lot like "nothing." But rarely will a leader openly communicate an answer in this manner. The thinking by other leaders, including members of the board of directors, will be there was insufficient or no material action invoked to avert the decline. This management inaction has several common causes, including:

- Denial: "It was not my fault."
- Victim behavior: "I could have done my job, if. . ."
- Piecemeal solutions: "I did my part." "Let's implement this part. We will work on the more complicated stuff later."
- Fear of embarrassment or credibility loss: "I cannot let them find out I do not know this. It could be damaging to my position."
- Incompetence: "If I keep quiet, they will never know I do not have the answer."

- Fear of job loss: "Regardless of the situation, protecting my job is job number one."
- Erosion of influence and control: "Everyone comes to me. I am supposed to be the go-to person."
- Optimism: "If we can just hold on, things will get better tomorrow."

Management inaction reflects a stagnant thought process. Progress is difficult when you are mentally frozen or moving in slow motion. If you are looking for a place to start, start with yourself. Start solving the management inaction problem by first being honest with yourself about your performance. Look inward and ask yourself the tough questions, including:

- Is the organization in its current situation because of my actions or inactions?
- What did I fail to do?
- Are there things I should have seen but did not?
- What could I have done differently to ensure a better outcome?
- What leadership and management skills are necessary to successfully avert a turnaround situation? Do I have those skills?
- What leadership and management skills are necessary to orchestrate a successful turnaround? Do I have those skills?

Once you have completed this introspective process, talk with members of the board of directors, medical staff leadership, and executive team members. Ask them candid questions about the current situation: Where do you think we are? How do you think we got here? And what do you think it will take to get us back on track? Have the courage to ask them about their impression of your leadership and management style. Look for repetitive themes and outlier comments from all of the discussions. Once you have sized up the situation, meet with your executive team and other hospital leaders to share findings, ask for advice, and map out plans for moving the organization forward.

IDENTIFY LAPSES IN ACCOUNTABILITY

The CEO or senior leader must focus on the desired outcome and navigate the process of getting there. A recurring theme with organizations experiencing financial distress is the lapse of accountability. These lapses can occur for many reasons, including the following:

- Team members are not clear on priorities, what needs to be done, and how to go about it.
- Team members are confused about their roles and responsibilities in the execution process.
- The organization lacks performance measurement systems.
- Leadership tolerates mediocre performance.

Identifying lapses in accountability starts with mutual agreement on targets and outcomes upfront. The next step is to apply time lines and milestones to the targets. Also, appropriate resources must be allocated for specified objectives. Everything should be in writing. Periodic reviews can ensure against surprises at the end. If the plans appear to be running off track, both parties have the obligation to initiate actions to get back on course.

Each turnaround plan contains goals and objectives for successfully navigating through the turnaround process. In turnarounds, you will not have time for discussions regarding performance appraisals or written job descriptions. Each objective in the turnaround plan will have a specific executive assigned along with a completion date. Individuals' and groups' performances are measured based on the completion of assigned objectives by the due dates. Defining and executing specific roles and responsibilities are the keys to success. Chapter 7 is dedicated to roles and responsibilities of each executive position in a turnaround.

Critical Success Factors Checklist		
CSF 2.1	To solve a problem, you first have to admit it exists. Acknowledge and own up to the problem.	☐
CSF 2.2	Management inaction can stifle progress. Identify and resolve the causes of inaction.	☐
CSF 2.3	Start the accountability process with yourself first. Be honest. Be candid.	☐
CSF 2.4	Identify lapses in accountability. Hold yourself accountable first.	☐

CHAPTER 3

Structuring the Communications Process

DEVELOP AN ACTIVE COMMUNICATIONS FRAMEWORK

Effective communication skills are critical to a leader's success, and the need for those skills is magnified in a turnaround. You do not need to be a gifted speaker; you simply need to be able to effectively size up the situation and answer the important questions in a context that people can understand. The following are the building blocks for creating an effective communication plan.

- Why do we need to communicate?
- What should we communicate?
- Who should be communicating?
- With whom should we communicate?
- How and when should we communicate?
- Common mistakes and pitfalls in the communication process

Why Do We Need to Communicate?

The primary purpose of communicating in a turnaround is to inform, educate, and persuade the key stakeholders to buy in to the process.

Successful communication can also protect the image and reputation of the organization and maintain or enhance relationships with key stakeholders, especially with employees and the medical staff. Do not underestimate the importance of effective communication in a turnaround. If a communication process is not well designed and flawlessly implemented, the leader's credibility and the prospects of a successful turnaround can be greatly damaged.

The purpose of communications is to obtain stakeholder buy-in, which is rarely achieved if leadership cannot effectively communicate what it is trying to accomplish and why. An example of an ineffective communication message would be leadership expressing the need to perform a turnaround "because we are losing money on the hospital's bottom line." In a hospital setting, some stakeholders may be motivated by this message, but many will not. Conveying the message in a way that resonates with a broader group of stakeholders while keeping your focus on the bottom line is possible. As an example, look at the same message stated in a different way: "The mission and vision of this organization allow us to provide incredible programs and services to this community. Our mission to treat the poor, our pursuit of excellence, and our vision to be one of the best hospitals in the country require us to consistently have a healthy bottom line. Your help is needed to continue our tradition of success." Joining the hospital's bottom line to its mission and vision will be more powerful than having the bottom line stand by itself.

What Should We Communicate?

The communication process starts with a message. The message should be one easily understood sentence that explains what you intend to accomplish. Clarity will be important. For example, "We are losing money, and continuing to do so will place the organization's mission in jeopardy."

From that one-line message, develop a 90-second elevator speech about the issues. It should contain the message followed by more details to make your case. It can also contain the mission, vision, and values of the organization. Be able to connect each of these to the desired outcomes in the turnaround. For example, "We are losing money, and continuing to do so will place the organization's mission in jeopardy. Our ability to serve the poor, invest in much-needed clinical programs, buy new and replacement equipment, modernize our facility, and stay competitive with our employee salaries will not occur if we are losing money."

Another example: "Our value of being good stewards of the resources we have been given requires us to be a fiscally responsible organization. To achieve this, we need to return to being a financially stable institution."

Beyond the elevator speech, you have to expect and be prepared to answer the following common questions from key stakeholders:

- Where are we?
- How did we get here?
- Where are we going?
- How are we going to get there?
- How does this affect me?
- What is my/our role moving forward?

Who Should Be Communicating?

The CEO or senior leader with the ultimate authority within the hospital is expected to be the point person during a turnaround. Serving as the chief communicator has important credibility and perception nuances attached to it. This responsibility should not be abdicated or delegated to someone else.

Keep in mind that a communication and public relations campaign should be developed and implemented for the turnaround process. This campaign will be addressed later in this chapter. A consistent message, along with talking points, needs to be communicated to the stakeholders and media. In addition to the CEO, other leaders can aid in the communication process. Chief financial officers can address financial issues, chief medical officers can address patient care issues, and so on. Other leaders delivering the message may include board members, vice presidents, clinical chiefs, department heads, and first-line supervisors. With so many individuals potentially involved, consistency of the message must be maintained through the use of talking points.

With Whom Should We Communicate?

The ideal response to this question is "everyone." In the absence of speaking with everyone, a comprehensive and methodical approach should be taken to focus on the most crucial internal and external constituencies.

Internally, four key constituencies are critical to success: employees, management, medical staff and physicians, and the board of directors.

Employees are by far the largest group to communicate with. Efforts to structure communications with this group should take into consideration delivering a single, ongoing message across the multiple departments, multiple locations, and multiple shifts in your organization. Communications with employees can take many forms: leaders attending regular or special department meetings; using employee e-mail blasts and newsletters; and hospital-wide town hall meetings.

The management group is not as large but is more complex. Within this group, careful attention needs to be directed at department heads, who are formally positioned in the middle of the organizational chart and therefore in the middle of the communication process. Department heads are responsible for the constant back and forth of delivering messages between senior management and employees. The department heads become the de facto human filters in the communication process. Even more, many department heads work with physicians and chiefs of services on a daily basis, such as in the emergency departments, operating rooms, laboratory departments, rehabilitation medicine departments, cardiology departments, and intensive care units. With so many touch points, ensuring consistency in message is important. This cannot be overstated.

The medical staff will probably be the most difficult segment to communicate with because of the presence of private practice physicians who do not spend a lot of time inside the hospital. Their main obligation is sustaining their office practice, although the success of their practice may run through the hospital. However, many opportunities are available to engage the physicians, including at regular medical staff department meetings (such as for internal medicine, pediatrics, obstetrics/gynecology, surgery, and emergency medicine), monthly medical staff committee meetings (such as quality improvement, care coordination, and medical records), and monthly medical staff executive committee meetings.

The CEO should prepare her own detailed notes about communicating with the board, but more important, she should take her lead from the board chair on how to work with the board of directors. The CEO should be prepared to make recommendations to the chair on the structure, content, and process of communications to the board. One nuance to anticipate is if the board chair asks you for your perspectives on certain board members. He may be looking for insight on how to deliver the turnaround news to different board members and how they might respond.

External constituents—the media, community, outside vendors, and past, current, and potentially future philanthropic donors—should also be part of the communications plan. Special care should be given to the impressions left with donors. Donors and repeat donors tend to contribute to what they perceive as winning organizations that can sustain themselves. The leadership of a struggling organization will need to confidently communicate a clear strategy of how the turnaround will make the institution more vibrant. This will signal to donors the organization is worthy of investment.

How and When Should a Plan Be Communicated?

Successful turnarounds involve well thought–out communication plans that develop transparency and define the situation before others do. Letting others define the situation can be problematic, especially if that definition has no basis in fact. Most public relations campaigns cover a consistent message, talking points to support the message, and a plan for delivering the message.

When structuring communications campaigns, consider the following components:

- Delivering a consistent message
- Supporting the message with clear and concise talking points
- Developing effective presentation materials
- Looking at all modes of delivering the message (from hard-copy updates to town hall meetings)
- Delivering frequent updates on project status (daily, weekly, monthly)
- Meeting regularly with internal and external stakeholders
- Creating information hotlines
- Identifying spokespersons
- Distributing press releases

In today's workplace, the use of digital media is important in communicating and connecting with your employees. Digital media—including e-mails, internal signage, closed-circuit television systems, blogs, social media, and smartphone apps—have several advantages over the traditional communications. Digital media offer an organization the opportunity to play both offense and defense. From an offensive perspective, digital media offer speed, frequency, repetition, and geographical coverage. Messaging can be queued to broadcast as a single one-time message or as a round-the-clock loop. A digital message can be transmitted anywhere in the world in a nanosecond.

From a defensive perspective, digital media allow the messenger to define—and consistently redefine—the message as the situation progresses. Communicating directly with employees also has the advantage of not having to work through an intermediary.

Digital technology should be incorporated as an ongoing leverage point in your organization's strategy to build an effective communication plan with employees and other stakeholders.

Remember to manage expectations during the messaging process. If expectations during a turnaround are too high, management will not be able to deliver and will experience credibility problems. If expectations are on the low end, serious morale problems can develop. Creating an even keel is difficult but necessary. You need to ensure expectations are in line with predicted performance.

Common Mistakes and Pitfalls

A true turnaround is a heightened situation. The pace of the environment will speed up because of the introduction of a burning platform, a sense of urgency. Elevated adrenalin levels can occur around this time, bringing about more rapid exchanges of information, analyses, and decision making. One of your challenges will be to keep the pace and settle the organization down at the same time. Invariably, because we are human, mistakes will be made. You should have a goal of minimizing the mistakes, but do not become crippled by them. The following are the top ten common communication mistakes made by leaders in turnarounds:

1. Concluding the organization does not need a written and structured communication and public relations campaign
2. Allowing someone other than the CEO or most senior leader to be the point person in the communications process
3. Not involving the board of directors in the development of the communications plan
4. Failure to create a consistent message with talking points
5. Not recognizing department heads are the de facto human filters in the vertical messaging process between senior management and the employees
6. Failure to use digital technology to enhance the communication process
7. Forgoing the use of external public relations consultants if the organization lacks communications resources internally
8. Underestimating the importance of open and honest communication
9. Not admitting mistakes
10. Failing to proactively reach out to all stakeholders

FIVE COMPONENTS OF EFFECTIVE COMMUNICATION WITH STAKEHOLDERS

One of the toughest things to do is deliver a difficult and unpopular message. In turnarounds, that is exactly what you will be doing. Many times, the message is something people do not want to hear but need to hear. Having a good communication plan throughout a turnaround is important for many sound reasons. At the top of the list is a leader's need to get most people on the same page and heading in right direction. (Note: You will never get all of the people on board.)

If you are a gifted communicator, you are ahead of the game. However, if you are like the rest of us, communicating skillfully is a craft you are still working on. At a minimum, effective communication processes in turnarounds should contain the following five components:

1. Preparation
2. Content
3. Organization of the content
4. A central message
5. Feedback

Regardless of who the key stakeholders may be—in your case, the board of directors, medical staff, and employees—the five components of the communications process remain the same. The change-up in communication is in the modification of content and message to a particular audience. For example, employees in general are first and foremost concerned with job security; physicians, with care of the patients; and the board of directors, with how the organization got in this difficult position in the first place.

The purpose of a communications plan is not simply to share information but to persuade. To persuade listeners that change is required in a turnaround, a sense of urgency must be developed that substantiates the organization's need to move in a certain direction. To accomplish this, you need a message that resonates with each of the various stakeholder groups. Sometimes, the same message will resonate with multiple audiences. Sometimes the message has to be delivered in different ways for different audiences. As the leader, you have to determine which persuasive message resonates with which audience.

Preparation

Preparation is the first step to establishing an effective communications process. It is also one of the steps most frequently overlooked. The preparation phase is usually overlooked for two reasons. First, the leader often makes assumptions based on his tenure and past experiences. And second, for sake of speed and urgency, he feels the pressure to get the discussions going as soon as possible. Making assumptions and moving ahead quickly without facts or information leads to mistakes.

There is no substitute for dedicating the appropriate amount of time to preparation. Start by gathering and reviewing the proper documents and information to ensure your discussions have clarity and focus about where the organization is. These documents should include:

- The current strategic plan, operating plan, goals, and objectives
- The most recent financial statements showing volume and market share changes, increasing labor costs, profit and loss, and changing cash position of the organization
- Operational efficiency data, including benchmarking and productivity data
- Quality management and clinical outcome reports, including patient safety goals and core measure performance
- Staff morale and satisfaction data
- Patient experience and satisfaction

Once your review is complete, meet with each of your executive team members to gain their perspectives on where the organization is and where they believe it needs to go. Next, get the pulse of the medical staff leadership. Are there similar perspectives or divergent ones among the members?

Content

In most turnarounds, leaders need to build a burning platform (a sense of urgency) as to why a turnaround is needed. The best way to get support for the platform is to start with the desired end result and systematically work your way backwards. Connect the need for the turnaround to the organization's and individuals' value system, goals, and objectives. For example, if the hospital is losing money, connect the need to stop losing money with the organizational value of stewardship or accountability. The need to perform a turnaround could be easily be connected with the value of clinical excellence from the perspective of "no margin, no mission." To provide excellent patient care, the hospital has to make money to reinvest in its people and facilities.

Organization

Conversations around implementing a financial turnaround can be nerve-racking, especially if you are a novice. Discussions between meeting attendees and leaders facilitating the discussions can become tense. Choosing the right tone is important. Communicating with the wrong tone can cause the discussions to become caustic, even among individuals who have known each other for years. The purpose in organizing the conversation is to ensure all issues are covered and negative feelings are minimized. The basic outline of talking points for this area should include the following:

- This is a difficult discussion.
- This is where we are.
- This is where we need to be.
- This is how I think we should get there.

This chapter and the remainder of the book contain excellent pointers on possible content for your conversation.

Central Message

In politics, you frequently hear members of a campaign team refer to "staying on message." Politicians use this phrase because messages can easily mutate as more people become involved in the messaging process. Leaders can also get distracted easily and lose their train of thought with so much going on. The most effective way to stay on message is for leadership to thoroughly discuss the message and succinctly commit it to writing.

Feedback

Make it a practice to solicit feedback from your audience. Getting feedback is the one sure way to confirm that your message is understood, even if your audience may not agree with it. Asking for feedback is also a way to demonstrate that you value their opinion. Reaffirm that you are all on the journey together. Do not be afraid to ask for recommendations. Do not be afraid of disagreement. The purpose of these discussions is to work through the thought process inside the room rather than in the hallways. If you are not getting feedback, something may be amiss or you may have a problem connecting with the audience.

You cannot lead a turnaround without an effective communications plan. Your supporters and stakeholders need to know where you stand and where you are going. Lacking a communication plan in times of urgency or financial crisis only leads to confusion and failure. Executives who believe they can finesse their way through the communications process—or be spontaneous and in the moment—usually have a short shelf life in a turnaround. Your hospital may already have enormous resources and great communications expertise within the organization. But if you do not have the expertise in-house, acquire it from the outside.

Critical Success Factors Checklist		
CSF 3.1	Develop an active framework for a communications and public relations campaign.	☐
CSF 3.2	Avoid the top ten common communication mistakes made by leaders in turnaround situations.	☐
CSF 3.3	Remember the purpose of communication plans is to enlighten and persuade.	☐
CSF 3.4	Remember that preparation is the first step in an effective communication process.	☐
CSF 3.5	Connect the dots from values to outcomes in the communication process.	☐
CSF 3.6	Develop a one-sentence message on what you are trying to accomplish.	☐
CSF 3.7	Develop a 90-second elevator speech that includes the message and additional details of what you are trying to accomplish.	☐
CSF 3.8	In a communications campaign, stay on message.	☐
CSF 3.9	Encourage and embrace feedback.	☐
CSF 3.10	Do not become defensive during times of disagreement.	☐

CHAPTER 4

Pivotal Discussions with Key Stakeholders

BUILD A BURNING PLATFORM

Chapter 3 discusses the need to develop a sense of urgency about initiating a financial turnaround. This sense of urgency is referred to as "building a burning platform." The metaphor reinforces the idea that action is required now or the consequences can be harmful. For example, if we don't quickly move to correct the organization's financial downturn:

- our financial security and existence are threatened;
- deeper, more difficult changes will be required to address the situation later on;
- our ability to provide quality care is compromised;
- our ability to compete in the market will decline; and
- our credibility for being good stewards of the hospital's assets will be questioned.

The right message (burning platform) can motivate the team to grasp the situation and work in unison toward its resolution.

ADDRESS THE FEARS OF KEY CONSTITUENTS UP FRONT

Hospitals contain a vast array of constituencies with different interest and priorities. The major internal constituencies are

- employees,
- managers,
- physicians, and
- board members.

Other constituencies include patients, unions, vendors, and the community. For this discussion, we will focus on internal constituents.

Financial turnarounds generate nervousness. This nervousness can give way to fear. Fear comes in many forms, including stress, uneasiness, or even mistrust. At the mere mention of a turnaround, individuals may first think, "How does this affect me personally?" Next, "How does it affect my colleagues?" And later, "How does it affect the organization?" These thoughts are the fear factor in high gear. The best weapon to combat fear is candor—be honest and upfront. A turnaround is one topic that should never be sugar-coated.

Understanding Employees

Job security is the first thought that runs through the mind of an employee at the suggestion of a turnaround. The personal loss of her job or the loss of a colleague's job can be traumatic. If their jobs are not eliminated outright, employees may be concerned about how their jobs may be affected by the change in the aftermath of the turnaround. Questions that may arise include:

- Will there be layoffs?
- Will my current duties and responsibilities change?
- How will this affect my department or service?
- Will I be reassigned to another department or service?
- How will this affect my tenure and retirement?
- Is this turnaround an antecedent to a hospital closure or sale?

Understanding Managers

Managers have reactions similar to those of rank-and-file employees at the mention of a turnaround. The immediate concern may be about their job security and how the turnaround will affect their status within the organization. Just below the surface, they are wondering who is coming and who is going. Creeping further to the front is a natural defensive posture to counterbalance the perceived uncertainty. As the CEO, you should not make any pronouncements about a manager's department or area of responsibility, especially in public venues throughout the institution. Early pronouncements can turn out to be inaccurate. Relationships can be damaged unnecessarily. It is highly unlikely that any one thing an individual has done at the middle management level would trigger a turnaround, unless it is of an illegal or fraudulent nature. What should be communicated to the group is that a comprehensive review process will take place, and they will be involved in the process.

Understanding Physicians

A physician's response to a turnaround may depend on his status within the organization—whether he is employed or in private practice. If a physician is employed, her initial reaction to the suggestion of a turnaround will likely be similar to that of rank-and-file employees and managers—anxiety about job security. However, physicians will also be concerned about the quality of patient care during this transition. These concerns will come in the form of questions about staffing, physician support, and hours of operation. Leaders must reassure physicians that quality of care will not suffer during a turnaround. You may even be able to argue that the care could improve if more resources are available for services because of a successful turnaround.

At the top of the list of priorities for private practice physicians is care of their patients. Being in private practice lessens the fear about job security, although many private practice physicians can be economically tied to the hospital in several ways, including through the volume of patients referred to their practice or through contractual arrangements.

As a leader, you will need to reassure physicians that the organization will be thoughtful and conscientious in its review process. Whatever you do, do not make guarantees about finances—you may be digging yourself into a hole you cannot get out of.

Understanding Board Members

Do not be taken aback if board members express some level of surprise, shock, or disappointment at the need for a turnaround. They are mainly wondering how a financial crisis could happen on their watch. In addition, board members are highly image conscious. Perceptions of the organization play a great role in board members' deliberations, as they should. Board members may feel they were negligent in their duties of providing adequate and appropriate oversight to management, and that they may have been able to prevent this situation. This view may or may not be true. The "if only" series may start here: "If only I had provided better oversight," "If only you had let me know earlier," and so on. When board members get through with the "if onlys," they will naturally turn their attention to you and your management team. They start wondering if you and your team are capable of righting the ship. After all, the current management team was the one at the helm when the hospital went adrift.

As CEO, you must be able to address the fears and concerns of the board, reassuring them you possess the required skills to affect the turnaround. Frankly, your job may depend on your ability to convince the board you can move the organization forward. If you are unable to convince them you are the right person, you should expect the board to consider other options.

CONNECTING THE DOTS TO RAMP UP FOR A TURNAROUND

So the hospital is losing money! So the hospital is having a difficult time! So the hospital cannot afford to do things the same way in the future!

What does all of this mean to the average employee, manager, physician, or board member?

Informing your stakeholders and getting buy-in during a turnaround is similar to the way you used a connect-the-dots book as a kid: The aim is to sequentially draw lines from one point to the next until a picture slowly emerges. In any critical situation, including a turnaround, you must get as many people as possible on the same page. Drawing direct lines for people that connect how their actions contribute to the organization's desired outcomes is a must. These connections help develop the passion for the work that has to be done and reaffirm to individuals they are still in the picture.

In a turnaround, connecting the dots and constructing a big picture is obviously not achieved by simply drawing a line from one point to the next. Hospitals are multidimensional entities with many layers of complexity. In these cases, connecting the dots will require more time. In the connection process, the goal is to engage the people and get them to truly understand why the turnaround is necessary, how they can help, and, if possible, how the success of the turnaround may benefit them. This is the classic WIIFM: *What's in it for me?*

Hospitals have many ways to use messages to reach out and connect to various constituencies. The following four approaches to structuring a message are common:

1. The Altruistic Message

The altruistic message speaks to a hospital and its employees' obligations to serve their patients and community. These two groups, which on many occasions include our family and friends, are counting on us to do the right thing. The hospital team should be reminded of these obligations, which strike at the conscience of most individuals working in a hospital. These obligations are usually in writing and can be found in an organization's mission, vision, and values statements. For example, a significant number of hospitals have a mission statement similar to the following: "Our purpose is to provide compassionate patient care to those in need." It is difficult to argue with this noble mission. It could also be explained that an unsuccessful turnaround could jeopardize the mission.

Further, most supporters believe the hospital should be the best it can be, a leader in the field. This belief can be found in most institutions' vision statements, such as "We strive to be a high-quality, well-run organization." If a hospital is losing money, this vision may be in jeopardy. If you believe you are already one of the best clinical institutions, do not fool yourself. You can still be better.

A final leverage point related to an altruistic message has to do with promoting the values of the organization, especially in difficult times. An organization's values are its core beliefs, which do not waver in good times or bad times. Hospitals commonly have values statements such as the following: "We have a duty and responsibility to do the right thing. Our patients and community are *counting* on us to do the right thing." These "right things" frequently highlight the virtues of being responsible, being accountable, demonstrating good stewardship of assets and resources, pursuing high quality and excellence, and acting with integrity. To connect the dots under the values of accountability and stewardship, explain that the organization should not be spending money it does not have, thereby causing the organization to go deeper into the red. This is irresponsible. The higher calling with accountability and stewardship should be to balance the books.

2. The Concrete Results Message

The concrete results message speaks to the managerial side of a leader's thought process. This message embodies a discussion on the importance of meeting goals, objectives, and targets. Most of the time, these areas are quantifiable. Some of the objectives that can be highlighted during a discussion of this nature include:

- Financial objectives (profit and loss, cash flow, balance sheet metrics)
- Operational efficiency objectives (productivity measures)
- Clinical outcomes objectives (length of stay, readmission rates, infection rates)

3. The Self-Preservation Message

The self-preservation message is about as straightforward as they come. This message is about job security. This message speaks to the need to make personnel changes if the environment and performance levels do not change. The ramifications of personnel changes can lead to a chain reaction for many individuals. Your ability to anticipate these events and the reactions to them will affect your ability to lead the turnaround. The personnel changes that might occur include departmental mergers, consolidations, or closures; terminations; lay-offs; job restructuring; and staff reassignments. Before announcing changes, anticipate the reactions and have a plan for dealing with them.

This message does not have to be negative; it should simply be honest. The hospital team must understand other options may be available before moving directly to job security concerns. Sometimes the turnaround can be accomplished by reducing supply expenses and administrative overhead. Sometimes it can be accomplished by increasing the revenue line, including reducing bad debt. But sometimes, if the organization is overstaffed and underproductive, staff reductions should be in order.

4. A Combination of Messages

In most turnarounds, communication to the stakeholders is a hybrid of altruism, performance shortfalls, and self-preservation. You must determine what to emphasize. The emphasis will depend on the condition of the organization and your perceptions about the current leadership and their ability to carry out the turnaround.

DEVELOPING A PLAN TO COMMUNICATE WITH KEY STAKEHOLDERS

Do not take your relationship with each stakeholder group for granted. When communicating with key stakeholders, take the time to think about what you are going to say. Do not assume that your relationship with the stakeholders allows you to be spontaneous in your messaging and communication plan. On the contrary, because you have this established relationship, you may have more explaining to do than you might think. For example, stakeholders may wonder, "If there were problems, why did you not come to us before it became a crisis?" The best way to approach the communication process is to work with your leadership and public relations department to craft a plan. Developing a plan for some may not come naturally. Take this opportunity to go through a brainstorming process with your team, attempting to look at the crisis and stakeholders from all angles. A word of caution: If a brainstorming session is going too smoothly, there is a good chance that major issues are not being raised. Remember, if everyone agrees with you, it usually means somebody is not thinking.

Board of Directors

Boards of directors, like the organizations they serve, vary from hospital to hospital. The primary differences are in leadership process, committee structure, reporting requirements, flow of information, and systems of accountability. These different factors play a significant role in how well the board can govern and how successful the organization will be. In times of strife, many boards adopt a back-to-basics mentality. This shift is understandable in turnarounds because many members seem to be confounded about how they got into this situation in the first place. Common sense would say they should have known, but in reality they are probably clueless. Common sense also tells us that when we do not understand something, we should go back to the beginning and work forward. Many boards seem to take this approach. Along the way to recovery, do not be surprised if you hear a member or two confessing they saw the car heading for the ditch but chose not to speak up.

Once confronted with the reality of a turnaround, the thought processes of board members become interesting. There are things they say, and things they do not say.

CEOs should anticipate the following comments and questions in the discussions explaining the status quo and the future strategy.

About the only time you will be exempted from these questions is if you are relatively new to the organization and the decline did not take place on your watch. But make no mistake—even if you are new, the board will be determined not to allow the same mistake to ever happen again.

A CEO's credibility is on the line. Therefore, be transparent and honest. Anticipate the following questions:

- **Where are we?** Clearly articulate the financial position of the hospital using financial key performance indicators, including profit, losses, cash flow, debt position, and level of business (customers) flowing through the enterprise.
- **Why are we losing money?** Break down the financial losses, including identifying what appear to be the contributing causal factors.
- **How did we get here?** Clearly explain the continuum of events and circumstances leading up to the current financial crisis.
- **Who is responsible?** Be thoughtful about who is responsible for the financial crisis. "No one" is not an acceptable answer. As CEO everything happens on your watch. The logical answer is you. However, extenuating circumstances may have led up to the crisis.
- **How could this situation have been averted?** Develop a short list of how the situation could have been averted. For each item, be prepared to offer specifics.
- **What do you believe we need to do to recover financially?** Use this opportunity to demonstrate a command of what is required to orchestrate a successful turnaround. This is your opportunity to communicate the high points of your turnaround plan.
- **What is our go-forward strategy?** Communicate how you think the turnaround should be done—and what help, advice, and support is needed from the board. Obtain board members' and board chairs' thoughts and concerns on how to move forward.

- **How should the turnaround process be structured and executed?** Develop a one-page outline for responding to this question. You will be asked this many times. Be prepared to explain how you can execute the turnaround plan strategy successfully.
- **What are the major obstacles to success?** List your top five and, as always, be prepared to drill down and offer possible work-throughs or workarounds to those obstacles.
- **How will we measure progress and success?** Make sure you have a quantifiable response to this question. Use metrics and mile markers.
- **How will this strategy affect the organization and its key stakeholders?** Keep in mind, the group asking this question includes your biggest stakeholders.
- **What are the downside effects if we fail?** Be candid. They have a right to know what the stakes are. If failure occurs, they will be on the hook along with you.
- **How will this situation affect the hospital's image and reputation in the community?** Do not take image and reputation for granted and give a knee jerk response. Put some thought into this. If you have a public relations expert on staff, work with her to craft a preliminary assessment. You can do a more comprehensive plan later.

Some basic questions the board may be thinking but will not articulate:

- What happened?
- Who was asleep at the switch?
- As a board member, have I really lived up to my fiduciary responsibilities?
- If we do a turnaround, what is the degree of disruption to the status quo?
- How will this affect me personally (image, self-esteem, higher self-accountability, increased time required)?

- You got us into this difficult situation—how can we have confidence you can get us out of it?
- Who will take the blame for this situation?
- Should we be looking at the competency of our leadership team?
- Does this situation require us to start over with a new leader for our team?
- Could this unfortunate situation be a direct reflection on me personally? On the board? On the organization?

At this point in the discussion, if the CEO and her leadership team still have credibility with the board, use the board in the manner it was intended: as subject matter experts, a sounding board, an evaluative mechanism, an anchor of support, a strategic resource, and a fiduciary agent.

Management and Employees

Remember that money is not the primary motivator for most hospital employees. Many of them, regardless of their position, believe working in a hospital is their calling. Despite the circumstances of this noble calling, however, economic reality does settle in. In turnaround situations, the reality is changes are required, and they will affect most employees. When delivering this message, speak in a way that resonates with the team and embodies honesty and integrity. The following four areas could serve as a basis for discussions with management and employees:

1. **Financial imperative.** Financial losses jeopardize an organization's ability to support its mission.
2. **Quality of work life is threatened.** Financial losses create conditions where departmental operating hours can be changed, employees' schedules and staffing levels may be restructured, and employee benefits are reexamined.

3. **Job security.** Financial losses require the leadership to complete an assessment of jobs and staffing levels because the majority of hospital costs are in labor.
4. **The need to reinvest in the facilities and people.** One of the first areas to feel the sting of poor financial performance is the capital budget. Reducing capital budgets is preferred over eliminating jobs, but cutting capital budgets can have its own drawbacks, such as not having the opportunity to modernize your facilities to be competitive. Not reinvesting in people means not being able to provide timely cost-of-living increases and not offering market-rate salaries.

Medical Staff and Physicians

Discussions with physicians and the medical staff may be the most difficult conversations to orchestrate because of their varying engagement levels. Some physicians affiliated with the organization could be in private practice, some could be employees, others could be independent contractors, and some might be joint venture partners. This combination makes for an extended continuum of relationships: at one end are physicians who are heavily tied to the institution economically; at the other end are physicians who may only have a loose affiliation with the organization, with independent contractors and joint venture partners in the middle.

Pinpointing the type of relationships will help with the discussions. The axis of the discussions with physicians or a group of physicians will turn based on the type of relationship they have with the hospital. Do your homework. Depending on the type of relationship, physicians will be concerned about the following:

- Employment status
- Retention of medical directorships
- Lease arrangements and medical office space

- Financial partnership arrangements
- Satisfaction of their patients with the hospital
- Loss of influence:
  - Discontinuance of prior relationships
  - Dissolution of positions and programs
  - Old players out, new players in
- Sacred cows
  - Clinical programs
  - Medical directorships
  - Hospital employees and departments
  - Office arrangements
- Staffing levels
  - Bedside care
  - Ancillary and support staff
- Capital investments
  - Facilities
  - Equipment
  - Programs

Regardless of the nature of the relationship physicians have with a hospital, they still have the shared expectation hospital administration will

- ensure quality patient care is provided,
- ensure the bidirectional flow of information,
- involve them in the decisions at the highest levels of the organization, and
- ensure operational efficiency ("the trains will run on time").

Some examples of talking points between administration and physicians during a turnaround for patient care and operational efficiency are the following:

- The importance of providing quality care
  - The use of evidenced-based medicine in the treatment process, including core measures and patient safety guidelines
  - Timely execution of patient orders
  - Medications administered on time
  - Tests and procedures performed on time
- The need to ensure operational efficiency
  - Respecting the physician's time
  - Maintaining appropriate staffing levels, especially at patient bedside
  - Ensuring scheduled ancillary tests and operating room cases are performed on time
  - Ensuring patient rounds are made quickly to allow physicians to return to their office practice as soon as possible

It has been mentioned before, but it bears repeating—the goal of communication is to avoid surprises and eliminate misunderstandings. Sharing information is more complicated if mistrust creeps into the conversation.

The Community

As CEO, you may be tempted to consider a turnaround an internal matter. This may well be the case, but it sure will not be a *private* matter. By the time a hospital reaches the stage of a turnaround, most people—inside and outside—already know your business, the good and the bad. From a public relations standpoint, you should lay the groundwork early to protect the public image and reputation of the institution.

Hospital leaders and supporters of the institution should clearly understand the proposition that the future flow of patients to the hospital will be based on perceptions in the community about the quality of care provided within your organization.

Some key pointers for you to remember when operating within the court of public opinion:

- Remain steadfast as a good corporate citizen, even during difficult times. Most successful hospitals have made it a practice to be active in the community supporting many worthy causes, such as supporting homeless shelters, the American Heart Association, the American Cancer Society, and many others. You may no longer be able to afford the level of financial support previously provided, so look for other ways to contribute, such as allowing your staff to volunteer at some of these agencies on hospital time.

- Invite the public into the institution so they can see firsthand the type of care being provided. Continue to allow the community to use your facility as a meeting place for various healthcare interest groups, such as cancer support groups, diabetes support groups, and lactation programs for new mothers. Set up facilities tours led by your public relations department. Take the opportunity to boast about the great services offered.

- Recognize the effect word of mouth has in the hospital selection process. Studies have shown that when patients have a good experience in a hospital, they tell three people. When they have a bad experience they tell ten people. Also remember that your employees are members of the community in which your hospital is located. And they definitely talk to their friends and neighbors about their work.

- Recognize the four most important ambassadors you have to the community: patients, employees, physicians, and volunteers. Recognizing that these four groups serve as your hospital's ambassadors is important. They carry the message that helps form the image and reputation of your organization.

Having them serve as ambassadors to the community should be a point of pride, and they can be a valuable resource for getting your message out.

Prepare for Detractors

When things are not going well, your detractors will start coming out of the woodwork. Do not be offended—be prepared. Seek to listen and understand. Do not attempt to discredit a detractor's position—your credibility can take to take a hit if you appear petty or vindictive. But do not be naïve. Develop a point and counterpoint document for the discussion, and have the document handy. Seek to demonstrate the strength of your position. After consulting with detractors, you may be able to win them over to your plan. If you cannot gain their support, you need to respectfully move forward with the support you have. If you cannot get the support of certain members of the board or medical staff leadership, your risk factors for a doubtful outcome increase.

Focus on the Patient

With all stakeholders, a purely financial discussion will not resonate. Ultimately, your organization is all about the patient. Position the financial turnaround from a patient-centered perspective. Freely acknowledge the organization's existence is not to make money, but to take care of the ill and injured and improve the health status of the community. Start and end all discussions with the mission and the patient. Be clear about connecting the mission of providing great care to the necessity of having a stable financial environment.

Critical Success Factors Checklist		
CSF 4.1	Develop a sense of urgency by building a burning platform ("If we don't act now, these are the ramifications of our inactions").	☐
CSF 4.2	Address the fears of stakeholders (employees, managers, physicians, the board) up front.	☐
CSF 4.3	Connect the dots to ramp up the process of initiating a turnaround.	☐
CSF 4.4	Get stakeholders to clearly understand why the turnaround is necessary and what their role is in the process.	☐
CSF 4.5	Ensure the focus of all discussions is from a patient-centered perspective—even the financial discussions.	☐
CSF 4.6	Prepare for detractors. Establish a legitimate point–counterpoint approach for the resistant individual or groups.	☐
CSF 4.7	Be clear about the end result and how the organization will get there. Be resolute.	☐

CHAPTER 5

Framework of a Successful Turnaround

GETTING STARTED: PREPARATION, PROCESS, AND STRUCTURE

Developing the right framework for a turnaround requires the right preparation, process, and structure. In a turnaround, good planning and preparation have no substitute. You must put a good game plan together before the leadership team takes the field. In the preparation phase, the goals should include:

- creating a clear understanding of the current situation;
- securing the commitment and support of as many key stakeholders as possible;
- creating a burning platform;
- establishing mutually agreed-on financial and nonfinancial targets; and
- establishing mutually agreed-on expectations, goals, objectives, key performance indicators, and key result areas.

In the process and structure phases, the goals should include:

- determining the composition, structure, and leadership of the turnaround team and subgroups. Energy and willpower are highly desirable qualities;
- determining the flow and management of information;
- determining the type and frequency of meetings;
- determining dates, schedules, and timelines: starting points, milestones, conclusions, flow and exchange of information, and important meetings.

STAGES IN A TURNAROUND

The prescriptive process of a turnaround has five stages.

1. Identify symptoms and causes (perceived and real problems), early warning signs, leading and lagging indicators.
2. Conduct a diagnosis (analysis) using tools and techniques.
3. Develop prescription plans (targeted action plans) that are hospital, department, and item specific.
4. Treat the causes (implementing solutions), the decision-making process.
5. Restore the health of the organization (reestablishing growth and vitality).

Stage 1: Identify Symptoms

Your goal at this stage should be to identify the causes of the problems. In this stage, remember to clearly distinguish between the *symptoms* of problems and the *causes* of problems. If you look at problems from a surface or superficial level, you are most likely observing just the symptoms. Many times to get at the causes, you will need to do a root cause analysis to dig deeper to look for answers. By the time the symptoms are evident, the institution's operating margin is already heading in the wrong direction. The days in accounts payable have risen, and cash flow has declined. These symptoms are fairly easy to identify quickly and up front. Symptoms are lagging indicators (see Chapter 1). In other words, they follow another event, such as a decline in admissions, loss of market share, changes in reimbursement, or a decline in image or quality of care. The real causes of financial decline are referred to as leading indicators. The leading indicators always precede the lagging indicators, but they are less obvious and are much more difficult to detect and quantify. Both leading and lagging indicators must be addressed, but it is extremely difficult, almost impossible, to complete a successful turnaround unless the real causes, the leading indicators, are confronted.

Stage 2: Conduct a Diagnosis

You should deploy industry-recommended benchmarking tools and functional assessments to more clearly understand the problems. Proprietary benchmarking tools are available for staffing and productivity; supply and purchased services costs; and statistical measures related to volume, throughput, and efficiency. This stage includes a drill-down process where problems are broken down into their granular detail. The granular level is where issues become obvious and the problem resolution process first begins.

Stage 3: Develop Prescription Plans and Targeted Action Plans

Based on the findings in Stage 2, a written work plan should be developed and shared among the leadership. Most turnaround work plans will contain voluminous information on the organization, including goals, objectives, action plans, dates, timetables, milestones, responsibilities, and affected areas by service and department. A section of the work plan should include the action plan. These action plans are drawn up at the enterprise-wide level, department-specific level, and item-specific level. An organization may have more than 100 action plans, depending on its size. The plans are highly detailed, containing specific objectives, dates, timetables, milestones, and responsible parties.

In this discovery phase you will use a lot of information to drill down into your organization's problems, eventually arriving at the issue that could be causing the underperformance. Many veteran hospital executives, based on experience, develop a list of possible causes and work through that list, sometimes using benchmarking data and other times using a process of elimination. Benchmarking data can be an excellent performance comparison tool because it is based on quantifiable statistics. On the other hand, using the process of elimination can be dangerous. The process of elimination can become a guessing game. This less than scientific approach can leave an executive standing in front of a group looking like an amateur at a critical time. Your action plan should be based on information, data, and conclusions that can be validated. Guessing and theorizing will not cut it. Make sure you get the approach right on the front-end process.

Another tool to aid in the discovery process is root cause analysis. A root cause analysis is a problem-solving methodology used to identify upstream events at the core of the problem. The root cause analysis approach should be familiar to most executives because it is commonly used in hospitals. One root cause analysis tool is the "five whys" technique found in the "analyze" phase of Six Sigma DMAIC (define, measure, analyze, improve, control). In this technique, you start with a problem statement, then continually ask why the team thinks the problem is occurring. Each answer provokes another "why" question to get past the superficial problem and down to the root level. Templates of this technique can be found at most Six Sigma vendor websites.

Stage 4: Treat the Causes

Your goal is to quickly implement the corrective action plan. Match identified causes with recommended solutions. Identify a responsible person and agree on a completion date that may include milestones. For example, if the hospital's overall labor and productivity indicators show the organization is performing lower than peer groups in a benchmarking comparison, the next step would be to look at labor cost by departments and cost centers. This responsibility usually is assigned to the chief financial officer (CFO). Another example is supply chain expenses. If your organization is shown to be underperforming related to peer groups in benchmarking, a next logical step would be to examine supply chain expenses and purchased services expenses compared to budget by department and by cost center. You can also examine expenses by vendor. This responsibility is usually assigned to the director of materials management / supply chain or the CFO. These are examples of items that would be placed in a corrective action plan. In both examples, the director or CFO would present, track, and report on the performance of these items to the senior leadership group and lead the process of performance improvement for these areas.

Stage 5: Restore the Health of the Organization

Your short-term goal is to return the institution to a position of operational and financial viability. Your long-term goal should be to reseed the organization with good management systems that will allow it to thrive now and in the future. Restoring the organization to good health will require a concerted and committed effort to make difficult and often unpopular decisions. Every team should draw on basic information. The most useful, easily accessed information available is benchmarking and best practice data. Benchmarking and best practice data are abundantly available through numerous public agencies, such as local and state governments, and proprietary firms. Data are available on a quarterly and annual basis for labor cost, staffing, productivity, supply expenses, purchased services expenses, administrative expenses, and financial ratios. Best practice data are available on length of stay, mortality and morbidity indicators, and infection rates. Market share data are available for competing hospitals, clinical service lines, discharges, and physician practice patterns. All of these data can be stratified and segmented based on location from a zip code, city, county, state, and national perspective.

MAJOR FINANCIAL IMPACT AREAS OF A TURNAROUND

In a financial turnaround, the value proposition is simple—get the revenues up and the costs down. Increasing profitability and financial viability without further impairing the organization is the immediate goal. Four areas most likely to affect immediate profitability and financial viability are:

1. Liquidity, cash, and cash flow management
2. Debt management
3. Cost reductions and productivity and efficiency focus
4. Revenue generation and revenue cycle

Liquidity, Cash, and Cash Flow Management

The most immediate threat to the life of an organization is not high costs or insufficient revenue. It is the availability of cash. Without the immediate availability of cash—whether in hard currency or short-term securities—an organization will find it difficult to make payroll and purchase needed supplies. The importance of this asset is easily demonstrated every two weeks when payroll is due. Any misstep here could have immediate repercussions on an organization's operations, including employee morale and the ability to keep the supply lines open.

Debt Management

Debt management can be a real friend to cash management in the form of finding ways to lower an organization's financial obligations as well as by simply reducing the outflow of cash. Some of the most common ways to manage an organization's debt include the following tools and techniques:

- **Bridge financing:** a method of obtaining interim financing that will be used to solidify an individual's or organization's position until more permanent financing is arranged
- **Receivables factoring:** a process of selling accounts receivables at a discounted rate to a purchasing company to obtain needed cash quickly
- **Extending payables:** a process of stretching out payments on current debt
- **Converting to notes payable:** a process of converting existing obligations into a formalized written agreement, usually between a bank or creditor, with a specified interest rate and repayment plan
- **Converting from purchase to consignment:** a process whereby a financially distressed organization, unable to pay for supplies and materials upfront, develops an agreement with the supplying company to stock the organization's shelves but only charge the organization when the supplies are used
- **Inventory management:** a process of controlling the ordering, storage, utilization, and quantity of supplies and material. A key leverage point, along with renegotiating pricing, is limiting the quantity of items and the time items spend sitting on the shelf.

- **Asset-based lending:** a process of obtaining financial assistance by leveraging the organization's hard assets. The loan is secured by the assets.
- **Sale of noncore assets:** a process of selling those assets that are not considered critical or essential to achieving the mission of the organization.
- **Divestiture of unprofitable businesses and subsidiaries:** a calculated process of divesting of financial entities and operations that may be adversely affecting the organization's bottom line

Successfully dealing with debt management requires significant teamwork on the part of the organization's financial management team, which may include some outside assistance and expertise.

Cost Reductions and Productivity

Cost reductions can have a much more rapid impact on turnarounds than revenue projects can. On the other side of the ledger, as an example, one common revenue strategy is to increase fee-for-service admissions. However, even if billing increases related to admissions, collecting the revenue could take 60 to 90 days.

The results of many cost reduction efforts can be seen almost immediately from a financial standpoint. Unless it is related to revenue cycle improvement, generating increased revenue has a longer uptake than cost reductions do.

According to many years of benchmarking, the three areas composing the majority of the expense category in any American hospital will be labor, supply, and purchased services costs. Labor costs can range from 45 to 60 percent of total expenses. Supply and purchase services expenses can approximate another 28 to 37 percent of total expenses. Most hospitals will find themselves within these fairly broad ranges. Because labor costs are clearly the major driver of an institution's expenses, managing labor should be the number-one priority. Most hospitals attempt to manage labor through some form of a productivity management system, whether proprietary or purchased through a vendor. Productivity management systems measure utilization of labor, usually by hospital, clinical service line, department, cost center, or specific position, such as registered nurses, pharmacists, technicians, janitors, or engineers. Studies have shown that the more profitable hospitals use less labor (full-time equivalent employee per adjusted bed) but pay their staff more (Safabi 2007).

Revenue Generation and Revenue Cycle

Organizations can affect the revenue line in two ways. The first way is to improve the billing and collection of monies that have already been earned. This method is within the realm of revenue cycle management. Improving the billing and collection in a hospital can have a profound impact on cash flow. Some examples of revenue cycle enhancements are improved coding of bills, renegotiation of managed care contracts, updating the charge master description, and reducing the days in accounts receivable through improved collection techniques. Depending on the particular area, some revenue cycle improvement results can be seen within months.

The other revenue generation method requires a more long-term perspective. This method involves increasing the hospital's throughput of patients, as mentioned previously. One way to increase admissions is through developing new clinical programs. Other examples of improving efficiency and throughput include timely patient discharges or improved turnaround in the operating room or emergency department. In the operating room getting patients in and out of a room is a prime measure of efficiency. The goal is to be able to accommodate as many surgical patients as possible. The operating room management staff should be routinely tracking utilization room-by-room, surgeon-by-surgeon, hour-by-hour, and turnaround time in between cases. In addition, the staff should factor in cancellations and add-on cases. In all of these areas management should be looking for barriers to the efficient flow of patients throughout the operating room. In the emergency department, efficiently moving patients through the system is just as important to the hospital's overall efficiency. Barriers to efficiency in the emergency department can start with a slow registration and triage process, unusually long wait times in the patient lounge, a less than timely caregiver assessment once the patient is placed in the treatment room, ancillary tests not done in a timely manner, slow results reporting of tests, and a lack of monitoring the process of discharging home or admitting patients to a nursing unit floor.

KEY OPERATING AND FINANCIAL LEVERAGE POINTS

Nine key operating and financial leverage points can affect a financial turnaround. These leverage points are not listed in any order of priority. They are all important and must be addressed.

1. Financial statements
2. Labor utilization
3. Organizational structure
4. Supply and purchased services management
5. Revenue cycle management
6. Clinical resource utilization
7. Medical staff relations
8. Physician contracts and medical directorships
9. Long-term debt

Each of these key leverage points must be carefully reviewed and surgically examined. At the beginning of the turnaround process, these leverage points can help you organize your thoughts and can provide an excellent guide to developing the written outline for your turnaround plan. If you are a turnaround novice, the depth and breadth of this critical examination might seem overwhelming. Do not worry. As you go further into the process and acquire more experience, the process will seem less daunting and complex. As the leader of the turnaround, you are not expected to personally complete the in-depth review process for each of these leverage points. Other senior leaders should be assigned some of these areas, coupled with their existing responsibilities, and be prepared to report back on their findings. For example, the financial statements, revenue cycle management, and long-term debt can be reviewed by the organization's chief financial officer. Labor utilization and organizational structure can be completed by the chief operating officer or vice president of human resources or both. Medical staff relations, physician contracts and medical directorships, and clinical resource utilization reviews can be completed by the chief medical officer. The most important thing to remember is that whoever is assigned the responsibility needs to intimately understand how his assigned areas function.

Financial Statements

In most businesses, three financial statements form the trilogy of the financial management process: the balance sheet, the income statement (profit and loss), and the cash flow statement. The same is true for hospitals. Other subsidiary financial statements can play a role, but these are the big three. Most nonfinancial executives tend to be drawn to the income statement first. Stop! Resist this natural temptation, and instead, check the health of your cash flow statement first. The income statement in itself will not reflect the immediate cash going in and out of the organization. Income statements are usually structured on an accrual basis, covering months, quarters, and years. You need to know what is happening with the money today.

The next step in the process should be to assess financial ratio analysis, such as working capital, current ratios, debt-to-equity ratio, and noncurrent assets ratios. You should be able to systematically work your way to these ratios and others fairly soon. But what you should figure out as fast as you can are the following:

- How much cash and cash-like securities do you have on hand? (Remember, the most important thing in a turnaround is the level of cash an organization has on hand to sustain itself during the financial distress period.)
- What and who do we owe (debts and payments), and what is due in the near term?
- Who owes us money? (Insurers in particular)

Labor Utilization

Labor utilization can be assessed through productivity management. Because labor costs constitute approximately half of all operating expenses in a hospital, giving them so much attention is understandable. Making adjustments in staffing will probably be one of the more politically challenging parts of the turnaround. The key to being successful in a political environment is to always remember to lead the discussions with quality of patient care in mind. This has to remain the priority, but you need good finances to achieve this priority.

Organizational Structure

Organizational structure can be connected to labor utilization as a topic of discussion, but it can also stand on its own as a topic in a turnaround. In assessing organizational structure, you should seek to identify inefficiencies in how the organization is put together. The key drivers when reviewing the structure are management layers, span of control, duplication of services, and overlapping duties and responsibilities. These indicators can be assessed on a department-by-department basis. If an organization is large enough—a multihospital system, for example—the assessment of operational efficiencies frequently rises to the hospital-to-hospital level. The goal is to get an efficient, cost-effective structure in place.

Supply and Purchased Services Management

Supply and purchased services expenses are the second-largest group of expenses in most hospitals' cost structure. Paying special attention to clinical supplies as you go through the review process would be wise. The availability of clinical supplies and vendor-preferred products can be a political quagmire for leaders in cost-reduction mode. For example, political issues can arise when a hospital wants to move toward a sole-source arrangement, in which the hospital receives a significant discount for providing a single vendor with more volume, or standardization of particular supplies, in which the hospital negotiates an arrangement to purchase specific supplies or equipment for everyone in the operating room to use. However, these deals may make surgeons feel you are limiting their options in the operating room. Ensure involvement of clinical personnel in this process so as not to get bogged down in politics of the supply and purchasing process. If the hospital has an operating room committee, this would be a good place to work through the process.

Revenue Cycle Management

Revenue cycle management is about legitimately maximizing the dollars hospitals collect and retain from providing patient care services. Other services may generate revenue, but patient care is the main revenue area. The revenue cycle management process operates along a management continuum that covers the preregistration process, registration, scheduling, clinical documentation, coding, billing, and cash posting. Leaders should pay close attention to the quality and accuracy of information obtained by registrars during the registration process. Inaccurate or incomplete information requires rework and slows down the billing process. The scheduling and registration process should occur prior to the patient arriving at the hospital whenever possible. Particular attention should be paid to the clinical documentation phase of a patient's stay in a hospital. This phase involves the accuracy and completeness of what is being recorded in the patient's chart by physicians, nurses, and other clinical staff. The documentation by clinicians will determine what services will be charged during the coding process once the patient has been discharged from the hospital. Whatever is documented in the chart is what the coders will have to work with in developing the appropriate morbidity level and diagnosis-related group (DRG) to chart patient and third-party payers. Ensuring the coders are properly trained for their assigned duties is crucial. The billing and collection cycle is critical to a revenue cycle operating well. The bills have to be sent out in a timely fashion, and the collection process should be optimized to ensure earned dollars are coming back to the organization.

Clinical Resource Utilization

Clinical resource utilization is a systematic process assessing the efficiency of patient flow, practice patterns, clinical outcomes, cost effectiveness, and service utilization in the delivery of patient care. Traditionally, it is a multidisciplinary process, led and staffed by a team from the case management and quality improvement areas. These individuals are highly trained and certified for their specialty. Activities involved in clinical resource utilization include examination of the following:

- Administrative denials
- Medical necessity of admissions
- Appropriateness of care settings
- Length of stay
- Cost per case
- Readmissions
- Discharge barriers

In a turnaround, all of these areas should be put under an intense microscope for assessment and improvement.

Medical Staff Relations

Medical staff relations are an integral part of a turnaround and crucial to the long-term success of the hospital. Physicians control the volume in every hospital, volume equates to revenue, and revenue allows you to purchase the buildings, equipment, and personnel to provide the care. Always maintain an open line of communications with the medical staff. Involve them in the decision-making process as much and as soon as possible. As CEO, recognize that you may agree with medical staff on the end result but not on how to get there. Develop a process with leadership to be able to work through difficult discussions. And above all, pursue a practice of no surprises. Surprises can damage trust and confidence between parties, although they may be pursuing the same goal.

Physician Contracts and Medical Directorships

Consistently laced with a heavy dose of politics, physician contracts and medical directorships can be an administrator's quagmire (getting bogged down in the process) or Waterloo (a career-limiting outcome to your decision) if not handled correctly. Leadership tends to experience more quagmires than Waterloos, but if a CEO does not handle a quagmire correctly once she gets into it, then it turns into her Waterloo. The advice is to develop a process to avoid either. A CEO should always involve her board in discussions when dealing with physician contracts. This is the best way to deal with a preventing quagmires and Waterloos. The more important thing to remember is not *if* you address this area, but *how* you address this area. Use caution. Use facts. Use your board. And use common sense.

Long-Term Debt

Too much debt can kill an organization. In a turnaround, some of the typical questions to ask include:

- How much debt do we have?
- Is it too much?
- Can it be eliminated?
- Or can it be restructured?

EXAMPLES OF DRILL-DOWN TECHNIQUES

Remember the old saying "the devil is the details"? This adage most certainly applies to turnarounds. Speak with anyone who has successfully completed a turnaround and they will tell you the turnaround did not pivot on some large project; rather, it was the culmination of numerous small projects and efforts that added up to a major impact on the fiscal direction of the organization. The challenge is how to get at these small opportunities. The answer is found in the use of the following management diagnostic tools. These are tools used by managers on a daily basis. Some of the following diagnostic management tools have benchmarking capabilities, while others are functional assessments of departments and services.

Benchmarking Comparison Tools

Productivity Reports
Productivity benchmarking data, which measure the efficient use of labor, can be obtained from numerous industry proprietary databases.

Physician Profiling and Care Management
By now, most hospitals should have electronic care management systems to support their case management process. These systems track physician practice patterns, variations in the consumption of ancillary resources (such as lab, pharmacy, and radiology), length of stay, and clinical outcomes.

Financial Ratios Analysis
This information should be equally easy to access and develop. Ratios can be obtained from the monthly and annually reported financial statements (balance sheet, profit and loss statement, and cash flow statement). Some ratios include the current ratio, long-term debt ratio, debt-to-equity ratio, debt service coverage ratio, labor to total expenses ratio, and supply and purchased services to total expenses ratio.

Balanced Scorecards
Most hospitals have scorecards. They are structured to meet the individual needs of each organization. Common performance indicators listed on a scorecard include financial performance, quality management and clinical outcomes, and customer service.

Functional Audit Tools

Hospital leaders often have functional audit tools sitting on the shelf just waiting to be used. If you do not have them, they can be purchased from proprietary companies. The audit tools include the following:

Management Audits

These audits look at many things, including layers of management, span of control, reporting relationships, and duplication of services.

Productivity Audits

Productivity audits are the leading diagnostic tool for assessing labor utilization.

Supply Chain and Purchased Services Audits

Because one-third of the hospital's expenses reside in this area, use of these diagnostic tools should occur on the front end of the turnaround.

Revenue Cycle Audits

Revenue cycle audits touch many areas. Seeking outside help for this area would be wise. At a minimum, if managers have audit tools, they can at least figure out where they should start in collaborating with outside help. Revenue cycle assessment will include looking at the business office, managed care contracting, accounts receivable, and billing and collection.

Physician Contracts and Medical Directorship Audits

Audits related to physician contracts and medical directorships should be done but done with care for two reasons. First, issues involving the medical staff can quickly become political and could and should eventually involve the board of directors. The only condition of not involving the board would be the size of the contract. With a small contract, use your best judgment. Second, the physicians represent the revenue line on your institution's income statement. Most turnarounds are not successful in the long term without the ardent help and support of physicians and the medical staff. Tread carefully but firmly. Many administrators have involuntarily left an organization because they lacked deft skills in handling the management of physician contracts.

Taken in aggregate, these audit tools weave a telling picture of the state of the organization. Never lose sight of the importance of the hospital's quality measures and clinical outcomes. These two indicators, along with medical staff support, will have the most profound effect on the long-term financial viability of the hospital.

EVIDENCE-BASED MANAGEMENT: BEST PRACTICES IN A TURNAROUND

The number of management tactics used to orchestrate a successful turnaround can easily range into the hundreds. However, not all tactics are appropriate for every turnaround. The use of a particular tactic depends on the circumstances within each turnaround. Evidence-based management (EBM) relies on tools proven to be best practices in particular situations. Exhibit 5.1 shows EBM tactics that have been successful for financial turnarounds.

USE INFORMATION AND INFORMATION TECHNOLOGY AS LEVERAGE

A word of advice: get well acquainted with information and information technology. In today's hospital, a wealth of information is at your disposal. Most of the time, it is right at your fingertips, including some information you may take for granted. Some of the basic information that can help you in your research and decision making includes:

Exhibit 5.1: EBM Techniques for Turnarounds

Cost management	• Freeze discretionary spending • Divest unprofitable core and noncore business lines • Freeze pension, 401k, and other contributions • Refinance debts • Eliminate nonessential services during nonpeak hours • Reduce average length of stay (ALOS) • Implement a hospitalist program
Revenue enhancement	• Accelerate accounts receivables collection • Increase upfront collection of patient copays and deductibles • Renegotiate unprofitable managed care contracts • Reduce denial rates by payers • Optimize medical records coding • Evaluate bad debt for appropriateness of converting to charity
Labor management	• Eliminate or reduce full-time equivalent employees • Eliminate or reduce overtime utilization • Reduce the use of agency staff • Consolidate similar or related departments and services • Cross-train staff • Reduce management layers and increase span of control
Supply chain management	• Renegotiate vendor contracts • Reduce supply inventory • Standardize the supply and equipment purchase process • Develop and implement a formulary emphasizing the use of generics over brand-name drugs

- Mission, vision, and values statements
- Strategic plans
- Market analyses
- Regulatory and accreditation reports
- Financial statements (cost reports, budgets, income statements, balance sheets, cash flow statements)
- Clinical and nonclinical department meeting minutes (monthly or quarterly)
- Vendor contracts
- Managed care contracts
- Quality reports
- Annual reports

- Productivity reports
- Patient satisfaction surveys
- Board minutes
- Executive staff minutes
- Medical staff executive committee minutes
- Prior consulting reports and studies

Information technology has exploded in the healthcare field with ways of capturing hospital and health information that were not conceivable ten to 15 years ago. More than 400 different electronic health record (EHR) products are on the market. Chances are you have one of them. Theses EHRs contain up-to-the-minute documentation on all types of critical information processes. This information can be stratified down to the nursing unit, patient, and physician. Another type of system is the computerized clinical resource utilization system. These systems predate the EHR and provide hospital-wide, clinical service line, and patient drill-down information on length of stay, case mix index, quality performance, clinical outcomes, and physician profiling.

Electronic financial management systems are also available. Many are excellent, including as part of their basic features accounts receivable, accounts payable, cash flow management, general accounting, revenue management, managed care contract tracking, and budget management. Some of these systems can offer modules in supply chain management and human resources management. Or these two areas can easily be found in separate standpoint software application systems. Some of the common information found in the human resource management information systems include information on FTE reporting, productivity management, segmented employee turnover trends, and employee benefits utilization and costs. Many of the electronic supply chain systems on the market have great capabilities. They can track utilization by type of supply, contain an automated inventory management system, produce cost ratios, and track vendor pricing and compliance with group purchasing contracts.

Most hospitals have these systems already available, and most of these systems can be interfaced with other electronic systems, making them even more valuable. As the leader of a turnaround, work with your executive team and determine what decision-support information is needed. Then work with the chief information officer, if you have one, and chief financial officer to get the information in the right people's hands as soon as possible.

Critical Success Factors Checklist		
CSF 5.1	In preparation for a turnaround, develop a documented structure.	☐
CSF 5.2	Use the five stages of the turnaround process to identify root causes of financial distress.	☐
CSF 5.3	Prepare and document a liquidity plan. Cash is king.	☐
CSF 5.4	Do not overlook addressing short-term and long-term debt.	☐
CSF 5.5	Assign turnaround responsibilities on the basis of technical expertise and individual resolve.	☐
CSF 5.6	Focus on the nine key operating leverage points in the turnaround.	☐
CSF 5.7	Focus on the diagnostic drill-downs into organizational details.	☐
CSF 5.8	Take advantage of opportunities. Review evidence-based management practice tactics early in the turnaround process.	☐
CSF 5.9	With the serious nature of physician contracts and medical directorships, the more important thing to remember is not if you address this area, but how.	☐

CHAPTER 6

Tools and Techniques of a
Successful Turnaround

PRIOR TO INITIATING a turnaround, a CEO will be confronted with three major challenges—time, technique, and tools. How much time do I have to complete this turnaround? How will I approach accomplishing the turnaround? And what tools do I have available?

The answer to the second question depends on the response to the first question. How you approach the turnaround will also depend on the institution's financial health. How steep are the financial losses, and how stable is its cash position? Depending on the answers, leaders can use one of two techniques. The first is to deploy the turnaround using a "hotwiring" approach. The second uses a "hardwiring" approach. Hotwiring is a shorter term, quick-fix approach. It can be accomplished in four months or less. The hardwiring approach is a highly structured and methodical process that takes about 12 months to complete. Most organizations use the hardwiring approach because the opportunity to connect the desired changes right into the organization's values system is better. To achieve that connection, significant engagement of the stakeholders is required.

Each technique has its advantages and disadvantages, which are mentioned later in this chapter. Regardless of which approach is taken, it has to be managed carefully.

Hardwiring and hotwiring use many of the same tools. If you are approaching a turnaround from a hotwiring perspective, you will use fewer of those tools because you have less time. Hotwiring has a heightened sense of urgency where decisions need to be made immediately. Tools used in a hotwiring approach are selected based on their potential to immediately impact the bottom line. Under the hardwiring scenario, all tools in the box are eventually used.

THE TOOLKIT

The turnaround toolkit should allow you to comprehensively diagnose and treat a turnaround. The 360-degree toolkit can be organized into three major sections: benchmarking comparison tools, functional audit tools, and evidence-based management tools. This type of toolkit will allow you to see all of the important metrics and how they affect the organization and environment around you. An expanded list of these tools can be found in Chapter 5. The tools in these three sections should provide broad and in-depth perspectives on the organization's operational efficiency, quality performance, and financial performance. The tools with the greatest impact on turnarounds will be those related to labor and productivity analyses, supply chain and purchased services analyses, and revenue cycle management. An overwhelming majority of the costs in hospitals is located in the labor and supply chain components of the overall expense structure. The revenue cycle management improvement analysis is where low-hanging fruit can be found. As a matter of course, leaders should opt for identifying the low-hanging fruit as a less painful alternative that can be pursued early in the process of analysis.

HOTWIRING: A QUICK, SHORT-TERM SOLUTION

If your institution is burning through cash to cover financial losses, and your cash position is deteriorating, you may have to at least consider the hotwiring technique. You may not have time to progress through a methodical step-by-step hardwiring process that may take up to 12 months. An example of a critical stage would be a situation in which mounting financial losses at the institution are posing a threat to the stability of its cash position. Here the threat is in the form of the hospital having to cover financial losses with its available cash, which may leave few funds left to address unexpected issues, such as major equipment requiring replacement or repair or significant damage to facilities. In this case, a quick fix is required. Instituting a hotwiring process does not mean a shoot-from-the-hip approach. Far from it—hotwiring a turnaround has to be orchestrated methodically, just like hardwired situations. The difference is in the steps involved in the implementation. In hotwiring, you will go directly to the areas known to have an immediate impact on the bottom line. A CEO should pursue quick fixes only after documented consultation with the board and leadership, which will itself take some time and require multiple meetings.

The major advantage of the quick fix approach is the speed by which it can stem losses. A major disadvantage of a quick fix is the top-down approach that can cause organizational whiplash when executed abruptly without much notice. Quick fix approaches do not allow much time for discussion or for employees to adjust to changes. If not handled astutely, the possibility of relationships suffering under this approach can be high.

A typical hotwire process could be as follows. A CEO would announce to her leadership team that the organization is losing too much money and the situation cannot be sustained. Each vice president and administrator would then go back and review his areas of responsibility by department and cost center, working with department heads and managers to determine how well each unit is performing based on budget and benchmark data. Administrators should look for underperformance in both areas and be prepared to discuss and make recommendations for expense reductions within two weeks. Shortly thereafter, the CEO should consult with the board about the findings and options. Tools to be used by administrators in this review process would include operating budgets, over-time utilization reports, staffing and productivity reports, supply and purchased services reports, and benchmarking reports. Once all of the above requested information has been gathered, the leadership team will convene and develop an overall hospital turnaround plan based on the research and findings.

When a preliminary plan has been developed, it will be presented to the board for review and approval. Some areas of the plan will not require board approval to move forward, including those that are considered a normal course of accountability for daily operations management. This distinction will be a judgment call for the CEO. Some cost-reduction efforts that could be implemented quickly to improve the bottom line include:

- Decrease overtime utilization
- Eliminate or minimize use of agency staff
- Freeze salaries and eliminate bonuses
- Consolidate departments or services
- Change hours of operations
- Decrease travel and meeting expenses
- Reduce dues and subscription expenses
- Decrease marketing expenses
- Renegotiate vendor contracts for supply chain and purchased services areas
- Spend down inventory levels

Consult with your board prior to implementing salary freezes, bonus eliminations, or department or service consolidations.

HARDWIRING: A LONG-TERM PERSPECTIVE

If your institution's cash position remains stable, you should still consider using the hardwiring approach, even if losses are significant. To hardwire financial improvements into the organization, focus on strategic measures that have a lasting financial impact, such as revenue growth and long-term debt reduction. Top-line discussions on revenue growth usually focus on reassessing service lines and clinical programs offered by the institution with the intention of developing a new program, expanding an existing program, or eliminating a struggling program that is nonessential to the hospital's mission.

The criteria for evaluating a clinical program should include profit and loss analysis and the program's support of your mission. Some programs will always be delicately balanced between the two spectrums. Hospitals should reassess their involvement in noncore services, such as owning medical office buildings, physician practices, and nonmedical companies. If these assets are divested, the impact could be reducing or eliminating losses or reinvesting the proceeds in a core program. Program proceeds from these divestures could also pay off debt or be placed in the institution's bank account. A tool that can start the discussions around divestures would be the institution's balance sheet. Use financial ratios to measure the organization's level of debt and ability to repay loans. Some ratios for this analysis would include debt service coverage, debt to equity ratio, and the interest expense metric.

One area of special note during a hardwire review process is the condition of the hospital's pension fund. Many institutions over the past decade have found funding and expanding an employee pension fund to be almost impossible financially. Seriously considering adoption of some type of pension reform may be helpful to the organization. However, handling pension reform can be another quagmire. Understand the differences between the two groups of employees when discussing tenure: tenured employees who are vested, and new hires in go-forward strategies. Pension discussions inevitably become complicated as you delve into the actuarial studies. Do not hesitate to reach outside of the organization for expertise on this subject.

The greatest advantage of hardwiring a turnaround is that it allows more time for the change process to be absorbed into the organization. Another advantage to hardwiring is that it allows a smoother, more effective communications process with key stakeholders. The main disadvantage is that hardwiring takes much longer than a quick-fix approach. But the added buy-in you may be able to obtain from stakeholders may make it worthwhile.

DEVELOPMENT OF TEMPORARY DASHBOARDS AND SCORECARDS

As mentioned previously, the pace in a turnaround situation is much quicker than the normal day-to-day pace of management. Because of this speed, keeping track of information and performance can be a challenge. If you already have dashboards in place, you are ahead of the game. If you are not using these decision support tools, developing a temporary set of dashboards and scorecards to improve focus and performance during the turnaround process will be beneficial. If you keep it simple, developing dashboards should not be too difficult. The temporary dashboards should track four important categories of performance information:

1. Financial
2. Quality
3. Efficiency
4. Effectiveness

For each of these four categories, a drill-down scorecard can be developed to highlight the details of key performance indicators. Exhibit 6.1 shows an example of a dashboard that can be used on a temporary basis. This temporary dashboard can also be extended into a performance dashboard.

Exhibit 6.1: Sample Temporary Performance Dashboard

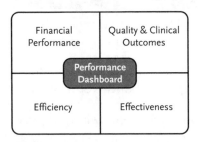

Financial performance	• Days cash on hand • Cash flow in/cash flow out • Profit and loss • Labor costs per adjusted patient day • Labor cost as a % of revenues • Supply and purchased services costs per adjusted patient day • Supply and purchased services costs as a % of revenues • Days in accounts receivable • Days in accounts payable
Quality and clinical outcomes	• Joint Commission core measures and patient safety goals (including: readmits within 30 days, return to ED within 48 hours, infection rates, medication errors, falls, and pressure ulcers) • Institute for Health Improvement campaigns (clinical process and outcome measures) • Leapfrog recommendations (clinical process and outcome measures) • Hospital Consumer Assessment of Health Providers and Systems
Efficiency	• FTEs/adjusted occupied bed • Nursing care hours per patient day: overall, medical/surgical, critical care • Turnaround time: operating rooms, ED, nursing unit beds, patient transportation requests • Operating room utilization • ED wait time • Days in inventory • Inventory turnover ratio
Effectiveness	• Profitability • Length of stay/case mix index/avoidable days in LOS • Market share • Patient satisfaction • Physician satisfaction

Critical Success Factors Checklist		
CSF 6.1	Determine how much time you have to perform a turnaround.	☐
CSF 6.2	Determine which methodology will be applied: hotwire or hardwire.	☐
CSF 6.3a	If using the hotwiring approach, look for ways to quickly improve the bottom line, such as reducing expenses for labor, travel, dues, vendor contracts, inventory, and marketing.	☐
CSF 6.3b	If using the hardwiring approach, focus on strategic measures with long-term financial impact, such as performing profit and loss analysis on all service lines and clinical programs; divesting noncore assets; and expanding profitable clinical programs.	☐
CSF 6.4	Early in the process, develop a 360-degree toolkit for the turnaround.	☐
CSF 6.5	Develop a temporary set of dashboards and scorecards to improve focus and performance during the turnaround process.	☐
CSF 6.6	Assess pension liabilities for improvement opportunities.	☐

CHAPTER 7

Roles and Responsibilities of Key Players

FIELDING THE RIGHT TEAM FOR A TURNAROUND

As CEO, the single most important task you will perform in a turnaround is gaining the support of the board of directors. The second most important task is selecting the right staff to execute the turnaround. Quickly fielding the right team requires accomplishing two goals. First, identify individuals who possess the necessary technical competence—such as in finance, quality and patient care, operations management, human resources, or information technology—to carry out their assigned roles and responsibilities on the turnaround team. Second, make sure those individuals have the right management skills and leadership qualities to inspire the team and organization and drive them to success. These individuals may already exist within your organization. If they do, you are ahead of the game. If they do not, move quickly to identify the talent externally (see Chapter 9 for more on using outside consultants). Regardless of the route taken, recruited individuals must clearly understand and embrace their new roles as change agents. A word of caution: Turnaround situations are not for the faint of heart. They are not a good match for individuals who struggle to make decisions. Selecting team members on the basis of personal relationships is unwise when past performance suggests the person may not have the skills to do the job.

MANAGEMENT AND LEADERSHIP SKILLS REQUIRED FOR TURNAROUND SITUATIONS

Common wisdom in the business world holds that there is a difference between leadership and management. This axiom applies to healthcare administration as well and has particular importance when fielding a turnaround team. Every member of a turnaround team should possess some basic skills:

Managers should
- Possess good organizational and project management skills
- Have a systems and process orientation
- Be data hawks
- Be able to read and interpret financial statements and statistical reports
- Be able to analyze staffing levels and productivity reports

Leaders should
- Be uncomfortable with the status quo
- Be results-oriented
- Be goal-oriented
- Possess critical-thinking skills
- Have good communication skills
- Operate with transparency
- Hold self and others accountable
- Be willing to make difficult decisions
- Persevere
- Be able to conceptualize, convey, and persuade others on ideas (based on the merits of the situation and circumstances)
- Be team players
- Be unafraid to take chances

TECHNICAL COMPETENCE: ROLES AND RESPONSIBILITIES

The minimum qualification for serving on a turnaround team should be possessing a demonstrated competency in a chosen technical area of management—such as supply chain, revenue cycle, productivity management, managed care contracts, budgets, or physician relations—or a known ability to be a good process manager. Knowledge of these areas is critical for diagnosing, analyzing, and making recommendations for improvement in the midst of financial upheaval. When assembling a team, include these core members at a minimum: a plan architect (normally the CEO), a plan implementer (chief operating officer), a seminal banker (chief financial officer), a guardian of quality and ambassador to the medical staff (chief medical officer), a patient care champion (chief nursing officer), and an employee morale champion (chief human resources officer). Exhibit 7.1 outlines each role.

ROLE AND DUTIES OF DEPARTMENT MANAGERS IN A TURNAROUND

In hospital settings, middle management is where the proverbial rubber meets the road. Senior management can design as many grandiose, sophisticated, and magnificent turnaround plans as it wants, but the success of those plans often rests in their execution at the middle management level. Most midsize hospitals consist of approximately 50 to 60 departments. Some of these departments have operating budgets soaring to $10 million to $20 million annually. The average 30-bed nursing unit could be staffed with 50 to 60 full-time equivalent (FTE) employees, including management and support staff. Department directors and managers control the lion's share of operating expenses in a hospital, and therefore should be actively engaged in the hospital's turnaround process. Do not work around the middle managers—work with them. Their support is crucial to the organization's success.

Exhibit 7.1: Roles and Responsibilities in a Turnaround

Title	Roles	Key Relationships	Questions to Ask
Chief executive officer (CEO)	Turnaround plan architect Chief communicator and motivator	Board of directors (particularly the chair) President of medical staff and major admitters Unions/bargaining units Employees Community	Do I know exactly what the problem is? Do I know what is causing the problem? Do I have the resources necessary to address the problem? Are the organization's key stakeholders aware of the situation? Do I have a plan for correcting the situation?
Chief operating officer (COO)	Turnaround plan implementer Productivity and efficiency czar	Vice presidents Department directors Medical staff clinical department chiefs Employees	How many FTEs is the organization using per adjusted occupied bed? What is the ratio of salaries, wages, and benefits to net revenue? How much of the salary dollars are in agency costs? What is the overtime utilization rate? How many layers of management and staff are between frontline employees and the CEO? What type of performance reporting system do we have in place to ensure accountability?

(continued)

Exhibit 7.1: Roles and Responsibilities in a Turnaround (continued)

Title	Roles	Key Relationships	Questions to Ask
Chief financial officer (CFO)	Turnaround plan seminal banker	Banks	What is the trending of our operating margins?
	Cash and cash flow top manager	Third-party payers	What is the trending of our expenses?
	Revenue cycle accelerant	Bondholders/bond trustees	What is the breakdown of our reimbursement and payer mix?
	Inventory and supply gatekeeper	Vendors	How many days cash on hand does the organization have?
			What does the cash flow situation look like—weekly, monthly, quarterly?
			What is our cash collection rate as a percent of net revenue?
			How many days are in accounts receivable?
			How many days are in accounts payable?
			What is the ratio of supply and purchased services expense to net revenue?
Chief medical officer (CMO)	Turnaround plan ambassador to the medical staff	President of the medical staff	Where do we stand in terms of physicians opinions of the hospital?
	Quality and clinical resource utilization point person	Medical staff clinical department chiefs	Where we stand in terms of providing high-quality patient care with good outcomes?
		Major admitters	Have the medical staff and its leaders been informed and engaged in the turnaround process?
		Informal medical staff leaders	Which medical staff members can be called on to support the turnaround effort?
		Chair of the medical executive committee	Where are the obstacles on the medical staff related to moving forward with the turnaround process?
		Chair—board of directors professional affairs committee	

(continued)

Exhibit 7.1: Roles and Responsibilities in a Turnaround (continued)

Title	Roles	Key Relationships	Questions to Ask
Chief nursing officer (CNO)	Turnaround plan patient care champion Key communicator with nurse managers and staff Patient satisfaction champion	Nurse managers Nursing staff President of the medical staff Medical staff clinical department chiefs Major admitters Informal medical staff leaders	What is the organization's paid nursing care hours per patient day? What is the agency use rate? What is the overtime utilization rate? Do we have quality issues in any specific areas to address? How is patient satisfaction?
Chief human resources officer (CHRO)	Turnaround plan employee morale champion Primary architect of potential staff downsizing	Employees Unions Department directors	How many individuals are employed by the hospital? Is the hospital unionized? Have there been attempts at union organizing in the last three years? Have there been staff reductions at the hospital in the last three years? What is the average salary of each employee? What is the average cost of benefits for each employee? What types of employee pension plans and savings plans are in place? What ways and mechanisms does the hospital use to routinely communicate with employees? How is employee morale?

The opportunities to engage the middle management group in the turnaround will be obvious from the start of the process. For example, one of the first steps in a turnaround is information gathering and comparative benchmarking. In this phase, information is usually gathered from finance departments, information technology systems, and the files and personal recall of department managers. All of these steps require the participation of middle management. Another example is analyzing staffing and productivity data hospital-wide and department-by-department. Middle management can be instrumental in this analysis of data and staffing patterns. Also, the key to understanding supply chain issues is to know the vendors, and middle managers usually know the vendors in their departments better than senior leadership does.

Once the right information is obtained, the turnaround team moves to the next phase, which is to make an organizational assessment based on the information gathered and using comparative benchmarks from databases in the hospital industry. The assessment phase can be divided into three parts: labor, non-labor, and operational efficiency. From a labor perspective, the turnaround team, including department managers, will examine departmental staffing levels, overtime, and agency utilization. On the nonlabor expense side, the team will focus on supply expenses, inventory levels, purchased service expenses, and contract services, among others. Collecting information related to operational efficiency may prove to be the most interesting. Here, the team will focus on management layers, span of control, duplication of services, overlapping duties and responsibilities, hours of operations, elective versus nonelective services, and the potential for cross-training staff.

The buy-in of the middle management group can be a major asset to orchestrating and sustaining a successful turnaround. Most managers are willing to do whatever is necessary to take care of patients and improve the financial health of the hospital.

Critical Success Factors Checklist		
CSF 7.1	Recruit the right team, especially subject matter experts.	☐
CSF 7.2	Clarify roles, responsibilities, and accountability.	☐
CSF 7.3	Include the middle-management team as an active part of the turnaround.	☐
CSF 7.4	Clarify and encourage an important role for the medical staff and physicians. Draft a one-page document in bullet format of how the medical staff and physicians can lead and assist in the turnaround.	☐
CSF 7.5	Assemble the team quickly at the beginning of the turnaround project, adding others as needed along the way.	☐

CHAPTER 8

Derailers: Why Some
Organizations Fail

SEEING SO MANY HOSPITALS successfully orchestrating financial turnarounds with their internal staff is gratifying. However, many more organizations are unsuccessful at the endeavor. Leaders and organizations that are unsuccessful in executing turnarounds tend to demonstrate personal or organizational qualities that, from the beginning, make it difficult to succeed. These qualities are called *derailers*. Derailers are events or attitudes that can cause individuals or organizations to go off track. Derailers can exist at the individual level and at the organizational level. Even the organizational derailers are often a result of some individual's shortcomings that have permeated the organization's culture.

The following are some personal and organizational derailers. They are not listed in any particular order or priority.

An individual can derail a turnaround by demonstrating any of the following attitudes and behaviors:

- Bad attitude or arrogance
- Lack of knowledge or talent
- Fear of job loss
- Inability to make the case (buy-in) and rally the troops
- Lack of credibility
- Inability to move outside of comfort zone
- Lack of willingness to make difficult decisions

Knowing yourself is the first step to avoiding derailment. Leading turnarounds is not the time to go into denial about your own strengths and weaknesses. Your fellow team members mostly likely already know your derailment qualities. Who you are, what you say, how you say it, and how you do things have been noticed and mentally documented by those around you.

A turnaround can also be derailed at the organizational level in the following ways:

- A poorly conceived turnaround plan
- Poor execution of the turnaround plan
- No sense of urgency
- Denial of or resistance to change
- Nonalignment of leadership
- Lack of knowledge and talent on multiple levels
- Failure to overcome deep-seated politics
- Long-standing yet counterproductive relationships
- Lack of credible and useful information and data

The question that always seems to follow these derailers is: Could something have been done to counter them? The answer is yes to some and no to others. For example, developing a sense of urgency and accepting that a change is necessary reflect a change of heart in how an individual sees the situation. This change can occur if an individual is truly sincere. On the other hand, some derailers, such as lack of knowledge or talent and lack of credibility, are extremely difficult to overcome in the short time necessary to complete a financial turnaround.

As the CEO, you should discuss derailers up front, during and after the selection process of turnaround team members. By discussing derailers up front, you may avoid them. Educate team members that these qualities could be influential barriers to success.

As a last word of advice, look to the collective qualities, strengths, and weaknesses of the turnaround team as a whole. On occasion, one person's strength can offset another person's weakness, and vice versa.

Critical Success Factors Checklist		
CSF 8.1	Know yourself and others.	☐
CSF 8.2	Discuss personal and organizational derailers during and after the turnaround recruitment process.	☐
CSF 8.3	Look to the collective qualities, strengths, and weaknesses of the turnaround team. No one is perfect. Recognize one person's weakness may be another person's strength	☐

CHAPTER 9

Internal Teams or Outside Consultants?

BRINGING UP THE TOPIC of consultants should not be viewed as a recommendation to run out and hire a consultant for your turnaround. Many organizations perform financial turnarounds without the assistance of consultants, and your organization may be one of them. However, the recommendation here is to carefully analyze your situation and keep your options open for success.

Key stakeholders will raise questions about who—starting with the CEO—is at fault for the organization's serious financial distress. In most cases, senior management takes a credibility hit for this question, regardless of the responses and circumstances. One of the worst things you can do in this situation is to start giving a litany of excuses. In your own mind, make the distinction between reasons and excuses. Frequent excuses include

1. it was out of my hands,
2. the market changed, or
3. it was somebody else's fault.

The solutions start with

- this happened on my watch,
- the following contributing factors have been identified,

- a plan will be developed and implemented to turn the situation around, or
- greater safeguards and monitors will be established with early warning triggers.

Frankly, neither reasons nor excuses go down well with your stakeholders. Leaders have to have the courage to step forward, admit their shortcomings, and own to up the problems and the situation. Correcting or improving a situation is hard if you do not first take ownership of it. And if you do not take ownership, your board may quickly start looking at other options.

APPROACHES TO LEADING A TURNAROUND

Leading a turnaround can be multifaceted, depending on the circumstances. Yet when the dust clears, you have four basic turnaround management options:

1. Using the current permanent in-house senior management team only
2. Using the current permanent in-house senior management team in combination with an outside consulting firm that will serve in a lead or supportive role
3. Completely replacing the current permanent in-house management team with outside consultants to manage and oversee the entire process and report to the board directly
4. Completely replacing the current in-house management team with a new management team charged with executing the turnaround

No one option is the most successful way to handle a turnaround. Organizations have been successful going with any of the four, depending on their needs, the comfort level of leadership, and the probability of success.

QUESTIONING THE SENIOR MANAGEMENT TEAM

Starting with the CEO, ask if each current staff member has the talent and resolve to make the difficult decisions necessary to get the organization back on track. A basic litmus test on the existing talent pool would be to ask yourself, "If *your* job is on the line (and it very well may be), is this person someone you can rely on with great assurance?"

The difficulty in conducting a turnaround with an internal management team has to do with the use of "hard" skills and "soft" skills in the management process. The hard skills are the quantifiable side of management, such as dealing with numbers, stats, and systems. The soft skills have more to do with the people side of management, and on many occasions, these skills can be more difficult to master than the hard skills. Soft skills—including trust, credibility, courage, and political savvy—are equally important in turnarounds because you will need them to navigate political situations.

Frequently in turnarounds, soft skills become damaged. For example, you may lose credibility in the eyes of some stakeholders because this situation occurred on your watch. Or your courage may be questioned—if difficult decisions had to be made, why were they not made much earlier to avoid financial catastrophe? However, the damage does not have to be fatal.

A CEO has five good reasons for using an internal team to conduct a turnaround:

1. To prevent a loss of confidence in the CEO and existing team.
2. To maintain job security. Self-preservation is one of the highest motivators known to man.
3. To retain control. Affecting flow of information and putting the right people in the right place is critical to success.
4. To manage expectations and perceptions of key stakeholders.
5. To retain the ability to positively influence the outcome.

A CEO also has five good reasons to support the addition of outside consultants to augment the internal staff:

1. If the internal team lacks the talent and expertise to pull off a turnaround
2. If the CEO's job depends on the outcome of the turnaround
3. If the need to make decisions and move quickly requires more resources
4. If the reputation and experience of an outside firm can be leveraged in difficult decisions
5. If the probability of success increases with additional subject matter experts

WHO WILL BE DRIVING?

"Who will be driving?" is a legitimate question, but it usually arises from fear—the fear of losing face and credibility, of losing control of the organization, of the impact on quality and patient care, of the effect on employee morale and relationships, and of community perceptions about the capabilities of the current hospital leadership. This fear can surface in many places, including with the board of directors, hospital administration, medical staff leadership, union representation, and rank-and-file employees. Engaging an outside consultant usually involves some loss of control, if only through the flow of information.

Remember, the natural tendency of many, including hospital leaders, rank-and-file employees, and physicians, is to ask whether the same individuals who got you into this situation can get you out of it. To lead a turnaround the answer has to be yes. And here is why. And here is how.

Some of the ways leaders can build the confidence of the stakeholders include:

- engaging them in the turnaround process,
- frequently communicating the status of the turnaround process to stakeholders,
- seeking their advice,
- allowing for input within reason and time limits,
- developing and sharing the turnaround plan, and
- being honest about the difficulty of orchestrating a turnaround and about your optimism for success.

USING AN OUTSIDE CONSULTANT

Sometimes organizations will make the decision to go with outside consultants if they believe members of the internal team are too close to the situation and cannot be objective in the process. Other times, the internal teams simply do not have the skills. And at times, leadership concludes it is more beneficial to get a fresh look at the situation.

If your organization turns to outside consulting firms for assistance, be thoughtful and deliberate in your review and due diligence process. First, determine what type of relationship and structure is most desirable. A relationship with a turnaround firm can be formed in several ways. The first way is a pure management consulting role for the turnaround firm. In this model, most, if not all, of the current management team is retained by the CEO, and the consulting firm provides subject matter experts in topics such as finance, case management, supply chain management, and revenue cycle, among many others. A second way is a combination of subject matter expert consultants serving in line and functional management areas, all reporting to the in-house CEO. The third way is to initiate a "turnkey" turnaround package operating under a management contract. Under the turnkey approach, the in-house CEO has been replaced with a new interim CEO from the turnaround firm. The new interim CEO will report to the organization's board of directors. Some current in-house leadership team may be retained with the new interim team.

Regardless of which approach is chosen, three areas of contract discussions between the hospital and turnaround firm are critically important: 1) the selection of the consulting staff, 2) the operating provisions of the agreement, and 3) what specifically will be accomplished and when. All of these topics need to be quantified in writing.

DEVELOPING A PROCESS FOR HIRING A CONSULTANT

If the decision is made to go with an outside consultant to assist the hospital leadership in the turnaround, the hospital leadership must obtain the best talent available within the consulting firm. Not all consultants are the same. Most of the selection process can be described as adhering to the basics and trying not to skip any of the steps. In his book *The Essential Guide to Management Consultants,* Michael Rindler (2002) does a masterful job of outlining how one should obtain the services of a consultant. Rindler not only addresses the selection process, he also goes into detail on how to select turnaround consultants.

Rindler (2002) indicates the first goal in obtaining a consultant is to create a short list. The short list can be developed by going through a basic request for proposal (RFP) process, which will later be complemented with a reference checking process.

Basic Structure of the Request for Proposal

Rindler (2002) recommends the RFP contain the following basic information.

Organization Background

The objective of this section is to briefly describe your organization, including history, scope of services, governance and leadership structure, and annual budget.

Problem or Challenge Background

This section explains the problem or challenge and why a consultant is needed.

Objective of the Engagement

This section describes the organization's objectives during and after a consultation. Further, it specifies the desired outcome.

Scope and Time Frame

This section describes the desired work the consulting firm will perform, the overall process to be used, and the organization's available resources. It also specifies the timeframe for the engagement, including start and completion dates.

Deliverables

This section specifically describes what deliverables are expected from the consultant, including reports, presentations, schedules, and so forth. In essence, this section should define the successful fulfillment of the engagement.

Proposal Submission Expectations

This section specifies a submission deadline, the format for the proposals, the number of copies needed, and a contact person who can provide additional information, if needed, and who will receive the completed proposals.

Selection Criteria

In this section, the organization articulates the criteria that will be used to select the consulting firm. The organization should specify the timeframe for consultant selection, including when interviews will be scheduled after evaluating the RFP responses.

Qualifications of the Firm

In this section, the consulting firm should provide a brief history and overview of the firm. The firm should specify what experience it has dealing with problems and challenges similar to those of the prospective client.

Qualifications of the Consultants

The consulting firm should identify the specific individual who will be assigned to the client and her specific expertise in completing the engagement. Special emphasis should be placed on the qualifications of the engagement leader. This section should also specify the number of references to be provided. Three to five references should be provided for each proposal.

Expenses

The consultants should specify their professional fees, any associated expenses, and the desired payment schedule for the engagement.

FACTORS TO CONSIDER IN THE SELECTION PROCESS

Many factors should be considered when selecting a turnaround consultant. Three of the more important factors are

1. the firm's experience and involvement in turning around financially distressed organizations similar to yours,
2. ensuring the right person, in terms of background and experience, is appointed as the lead consultant on the project, and
3. the firm's willingness to commit to specific dates, timetables, and mile markers related to the completion of the project.

PITFALLS TO AVOID

Hospital leadership should avoid four common pitfalls in selecting and working with turnaround firms—or any consulting firms for that matter. The first pitfall is conducting a superficial evaluation process in which adequate due diligence is not properly completed because of perceived time constraints. A second pitfall, and related to the first, is to avoid selecting a turnaround firm solely based on reputation. Third, after the turnaround is underway, is terminating the services of *all* of the hospital's top management at the same time and replacing them with interim executives from the firm. Doing so may lead to the fourth pitfall, which is becoming overly dependent on the consulting firm. If the decision is made to sever all or part of the senior leadership team, the exit process should be incremental to guard against abrupt and mass loss of institutional memory and critical information.

Critical Success Factors Checklist		
CSF 9.1	Do not give excuses—give solutions!	☐
CSF 9.2	Be honest with yourself and your team.	☐
CSF 9.3	Decide whether the internal leadership team has the ability to execute the turnaround. (Decide based on competence, not personal comfort.)	☐
CSF 9.4	If outside consultants are brought in to assist you in the turnaround, determine up front who will be doing the driving.	☐
CSF 9.5	Act with confidence.	☐

CHAPTER 10

Special Considerations

CONDUCTING A TURNAROUND is difficult in itself. But for certain organizations, turnarounds can have added dimensions that can present challenges. These added dimensions must be taken into consideration to ensure a good outcome. This chapter examines four types of organizations that can present additional challenges and identifies four particular areas that must be considered when these organizations undergo a turnaround.

In earlier chapters, I highlight the multiple stakeholders—such as the board of directors, senior management, middle management, employees, medical staff, and patients—and other issues present in most turnarounds. In most turnarounds, the organization has one board of directors, one senior management group, and one set of mission, vision, and values statements. However, some turnarounds have to be orchestrated in highly complex and diverse environments with even more moving parts. These moving parts are the heterogeneous factors that must be woven together into a cohesive, shared sense of purpose about achieving a successful turnaround. The following organizations are classic examples of these diverse environments and the presence of heterogeneous factors and stakeholder interests beyond what you might find in the average community hospital.

- Academic medical centers
- Faith-based institutions

- Public entities (county, city, or district)
- For-profit entities

Also, the situation can be even more complicated because some organizations can have more than one characteristic described in this list. For example, an academic medical center could also be a faith-based organization and public entity or safety net institution. Further, a faith-based organization could be owned by a for-profit entity. And a safety net institution could easily be part of a multi-hospital system. These varying characteristics make for a dynamic environment.

Some of the more important heterogeneous factors and added challenges to take into consideration for the above organizations include:

- Additional stakeholders, decision makers, and influencers of decisions
- Alignment of missions, visions, and values
- Financial objectives and multiple funding sources
- Alignment of priorities (at each level of leadership)

ACADEMIC MEDICAL CENTERS

Academic medical centers (AMC) are usually rich in tradition, depth and breadth of clinical expertise, and in the introduction of other stakeholders. In fact, of all diverse organizations, AMCs probably have the most potential for layering and the presence of additional key stakeholders. This layering is caused by a number of factors, including hospital ownership and reporting relationships. For example, a hospital owned by a university could be a legally separate entity reporting to a hospital or AMC board, or it could report to the dean of the medical school or the CEO of the medical center. The legal and reporting structure will affect how priorities are listed and how decisions will be made.

Additional Stakeholders, Decision Makers, and Influencers

Additional stakeholders in an academic environment include the following:

- Vice presidents of health affairs
- Medical school deans
- Medical school clinical department chiefs or chairs
- Clinical faculty and star clinical faculty with excellent reputations
- Faculty practice plan participants (physician compensation)
- Hospital or medical center boards of directors
- University presidents (for university-owned hospitals)
- University boards of directors (for university-owned hospitals)

Mission, Vision, and Values

For purposes of this discussion, assume a hospital and the AMC as a whole are in alignment on the vision and values. Depending on the organizational ownership, structure, and reporting relationship, the mission (purpose) is often the same for both organizations. But it may be different at times. Many traditional AMCs' tripod mission of education, research, and service have been agreed to by the medical school and hospital. Most interested parties would agree this mission is appropriate for the entire academic enterprise. Difficulty arises in where the emphasis is placed. Which leg of the tripod mission will take priority? Or will all three have equal weight? The medical school believes education and research are critical to its success, although continued declining school revenues have given medical schools an added appreciation for the (patient) service revenue flowing through their departmental budgets. Teaching hospitals, on the other hand, tend to place a high priority on service revenue as the life blood for keeping the hospital and clinical enterprise afloat. When an AMC is in a turnaround, the hospital leadership must convince its academic brethren that service revenue has to be a heightened priority if the clinical enterprise is to survive.

Financial Objectives and Multiple Funding Sources

How the money flows through the hospital and AMC is also important. In most private, not-for-profit institutions, the most common flow of dollars into a hospital is through insurance payers as a result of providing patient care. These payers usually include commercial insurance, Medicare, and Medicaid. In an academic environment, these three sources of revenue are also present and listed under service revenue. But AMCs have three other funding sources that could have some bearing on the financial health of the hospital—tuition, research grants, and philanthropy. Together with service revenue, these are the four primary revenue sources for most AMCs. Chances are practically nonexistent that the hospital will be receiving any portion of tuition dollars. These go directly to the university and medical school. But the distribution and flow of research grants and philanthropy dollars could be different. Dollars in these two buckets could flow to the hospital's operating and capital budgets as restricted or unrestricted funds. An example of research grants in the hospital setting includes significant grants for translational research conducted at the patient's bedside as a result of bench research completed in the lab at the medical school. Other than service revenue, the allocation and flow of research grants and dollars would be the high impact financial area in an AMC. (Faculty practice plan revenue has been excluded from this discussion.)

Alignment of Priorities

The three major spokes in the wheel of an AMC are the university (president and board of directors), the medical school (dean, chairs, and faculty), and the hospital (CEO and leadership team). The development of priorities should be in response to the size of the hospital's deficit. If the situation is urgent, deference should be given to the hospital and its priorities, at least until the crisis has abated. If the situation is less ominous from a financial perspective, then other stakeholders' concerns should play a more prominent role in the development of the turnaround priorities.

FAITH-BASED INSTITUTIONS

Most religious healthcare institutions in the United States fall into one of two categories: Protestant (Baptist, Methodist, and Presbyterian) or Catholic. Over the past several decades, many religious hospital organizations have fallen into financially dire straits. That many of these institutions find themselves in financial difficulty is not surprising. Religious leaders have a laser focus on the mission of the hospital that comes with years training. The articulated mission of many religious hospital organizations is to be highly inclusive, promoting exemplary community outreach programs and providing care regardless of ability to pay. When the passion for such a noble mission outweighs the availability of resources, financial issues can surface. In the end, someone has to pay or things come to a halt. A balance has to be achieved between what is desirable and what is affordable.

Additional Stakeholders, Decision Makers, and Influencers

Since the 1980s, religious institutions have gone through tremendous transformations. They have organized, reorganized, restructured, consolidated, and expanded on a level akin to a *Fortune* 500 company. Creating holding companies, parent companies, subsidiaries, and sister companies has all been part of the effort to position the institutions to be more competitive in the market. An interesting by-product of this corporate reorganization has been the creation of layers of leadership and organizational structures, such as local ministries, regional offices, national corporate offices, and sponsors. Depending on the severity of the financial situation, local CEOs will need to engage these stakeholder leaders directly or indirectly through higher-level management. The degree of involvement will probably be determined in the process of the discussing the topic of leadership.

Mission, Vision, and Values

The mission, vision, and values of religious healthcare organizations have been visible in the United States for centuries and have been nurtured and grown with the support of religious sponsors. For these organizations, their identity is confirmed by their mission, which has its origins in the pursuit of the healing mission of Christ. But nowhere is the old adage "no margin, no mission" more applicable than in the religious healthcare environment. From the corporate office with the support of the sponsors down to the local ministries, these organizations must ask themselves how much mission they can afford.

Financial Objectives and Multiple Funding Sources

When religious organizations started to go through corporate transformations, they began to invoke more financial discipline and accountability in their management systems and processes. This change means that today you can go to just about any religious healthcare organization, at any level, and find a concrete financial management plan in place. The difficulty arises in sticking with the plan when internal and external forces seem to be going in different directions. For local ministries, a safety mechanism called a "corporate allocation" can save the day. In a corporate allocation, the corporate office of the religious group that owns the hospital intercedes and covers the financial shortfall of the distressed institution. But this is a "break the glass and a pull the lever only as a last resort" option. Keeping the many layers of leadership involved in the discussion about the financial health of the hospital, especially during a financially distressed times, is critical.

Alignment of Priorities

Alignment of priorities in a religious organization can involve a moral discussion just as much as a financial one. Today, most religious healthcare organizations have developed a common leadership framework that spans all levels, from local ministries and regional offices to corporate and national offices. These frameworks help set priorities from a hierarchical and horizontal perspective. Organizational goals and objectives are developed at the beginning of the year and monitored on a monthly basis, if not more frequently. From a financial perspective, one of the common values around which goals are created is stewardship. Stewardship at its essence is the wise use of limited resources, given to support the mission and vision of the organization. If a local ministry is in a turnaround, a good starting point for ensuring alignment would be to refer to the common leadership framework.

PUBLIC ENTITIES

Public health and hospital systems have a long and distinguished place in history as humanitarian benefactors to our society in times of great need. Throughout this country's history, public hospitals have consistently served as the last bastion and protector of those in need. Public hospitals and health systems serve as society's healthcare safety net; without them, many lives would be lost to preventable injuries, illnesses, and diseases. However, this noble mission is not provided to society without costs and constraints. These constraints usually correlate to the ownership of the public entity. Most public hospitals are owned by a governmental entity, such as a city, county, or hospital district. In these structures, healthcare is very much a local business and a political institution.

Additional Stakeholders, Decision Makers, and Influencers

Over time, public hospitals have evolved to be fairly similar to other hospitals in the field from an internal management perspective. The exterior oversight is where key differences come into focus. Public hospitals are ultimately accountable to the local taxpayers, who serve as a significant part of their funding base in most instances. This accountability to the taxpayers is discharged through duly elected or appointed officials who provide oversight. These officials can include

- an elected city or county mayor,
- an appointed county executive,
- an elected city council or county commission, or
- a hospital district board enacted through state statues.

Regardless of the public structure, politics play a significant role in the decision-making process in public hospitals. Failure to recognize this dimension can be costly to an institution in time and money. CEOs should develop a list of key stakeholders upfront. The list may be long and therefore not easy to manage. If you think the stakeholders list is too long, vet the list and shorten it by consulting with trusted advisors, such as members of your executive team.

Mission, Vision, and Values

In addition to the public hospital's own mission, the mission and vision of a larger public governing body may also exist. Elected or appointed political leaders and their involvement in the affairs of public hospitals may be ever present in a hospital administrator's thought process. The first thought invariably is for the budgets—one for the hospital itself and one for the agency that has legal oversight of the hospital and its assets, such as a county or city government. In many cases, the state government also factors into the equation for related annual Medicaid budgets and reimbursement. A second area for the public hospital administrator to ponder is the level of services the hospital offers to the community. The level of services offered can affect the finances of the institution. As an example, if the institution offers high-risk obstetrical services, burn services, neonatal services, or trauma services, these specialties each have a cost attached to them. Political discussions and implications have to be factored into any equation regarding public hospital finances and the potential execution of a financial turnaround.

Financial Objectives and Multiple Funding Sources

From a political perspective, public hospitals are frequently viewed in narrow terms, either as an asset or a liability. If the hospital is viewed as a liability, it is usually for financial reasons. Viewed through the lenses of politicians, does the financial instability of the hospital jeopardize the larger (parent) governmental entity, such as the city, county, district, state, or some other political body? Will the financial instability affect bond ratings, current funding levels, clinical services available to the public, and equally important, will it affect you personally?

Alignment of Priorities

Deft public hospital leadership is required to ensure alignment of priorities from the top to the bottom of the political process. Navigating this political process is an added challenge of operating within the public hospital domain. Alignment of priorities is crucial to success and moving forward. Not getting most players on the same page can hamper progress, and in some instances, prove fatal. One of the best tools for achieving alignment in a political environment is to plan ahead and start to build coalitions for the plans early in the process.

FOR-PROFIT ENTITIES

About 10 percent of the nation's hospitals are classified as investor owned, which means for profit. Once seen as the pariahs of the hospital industry, for-profit hospitals have become mainstream and are now emulated by many not-for-profit hospital systems. In most instances, for-profit hospitals have proven to be capable of carrying out a societal mission of clinical service to the community while simultaneously maintaining a laser-like focus on the bottom line. And so it bears repeating here: Even though, clinically speaking, some of the best hospitals in the country are owned by for-profits, for-profit hospitals are in business to make money.

Additional Stakeholders, Decision Makers, and Influencers

Similar to their public hospital and religious hospital counterparts, for-profit hospitals have quite a few stakeholders outside the four walls of the institution. First, they have regional and divisional executives who have been assigned ultimate responsibility for the hospital's performance. Second, corporate executives, including the corporate officers, report performance on a quarterly basis in a public forum. And third, public investors provide the company with the necessary capital and financing.

Mission, Vision, and Values

When examining for-profit hospitals, the visions and values are fairly similar to those of not-for-profit hospitals. The organizations aspire to be greater than they are today. They tend to have all of the same intangible values as not-for-profits, with the exception of a heavier emphasis on stewardship. For-profits have acquitted themselves well on the clinical side with service to the community. However, a for-profit hospital company's purpose is return on investment and profits. The expectations in these areas are clearly articulated. If the financial returns are not there as promised, the capital markets will dry up and disappear.

Financial Objectives and Multiple Funding Sources

Most for-profit hospital systems get their funding from the public capital markets through the sale of stock. Every day, individuals and companies purchase the stock of these hospital companies with the expectation that they will be rewarded with higher returns later. As they do with most other publicly traded companies, these investors keep tabs on a company's performance and their stocks through quarterly reporting processes to the public. These investors can be hawkish when performance does not line up with expectations. Most for-profit hospital companies are organized in a multihospital system with regions, divisions, and a corporate office and leadership group. The financial incentives of the corporate office CEO down to hospital department directors are aligned to produce a positive operating margin. When this does not occur, the train comes to a halt, and a serious self-examination commences.

Alignment of Priorities

If a local for-profit hospital is off target with any performance indicators, whether financial or nonfinancial, the hospital CEO and her team have to expect lightning-speed questions from the leadership at the regional or divisional level.

In conclusion, some organizations, based on ownership characteristics, can present additional challenges in the turnaround process. A CEO's success in orchestrating a turnaround may well depend on her ability to recognize the different traits that come with different types of ownership, using the four-point framework: additional stakeholders, decision makers, and influencers; mission, vision, and values; financial objectives and multiple funding sources; and aligning priorities.

Initially, a CEO may want to develop the four-point framework on her own. However, a better outcome may be achieved with greater input from colleagues, trusted advisors, and key stakeholders. If discussions with stakeholders are not going your way, do not take it personally. It is probably just business (or politics). Take a step back and quickly reassess the situation and environment. Look for signs that you may be overlooking something. Also, reexamine the development and execution of your communications plan. Is the plan structured in a manner to effectively achieve buy-in into the turnaround process? Is your message resonating with stakeholders? Document discussions and observations to help with the thought and examination process.

Critical Success Factors Checklist		
CSF 10.1	Not all hospitals are the same. Consider the type of organization requiring turnaround.	☐
CSF 10.2	The basics of the turnaround plan you develop will be similar, but recognize the many nuances of your plan based on the organization's ownership status.	☐
CSF 10.3	Make a list of stakeholders to prevent overlooking anyone. Once the list is developed, start narrowing the list based on time, required resources, and politics.	☐
CSF 10.4	Academic medical centers tend to have a longer list of local stakeholders due to the possible university, medical school, and faculty practice connections. This can be complicated even further if the institution is publicly owned.	☐
CSF 10.5	Be aware that for-profit hospitals have an extremely low tolerance for financial losses. Be prepared to move quickly or be moved quickly.	☐
CSF 10.6	If discussions with stakeholders are not going your way, do not take it personally. It is probably just business (or politics). Take a step back and quickly reassess the situation and environment. Look for signs you may be overlooking something and falling short in the communications process.	☐

CHAPTER 11

Operating in the Post-Turnaround Era

CREATING CLOSURE

Your organization has accomplished much during the turnaround phase. These accomplishments should be celebrated openly and with great thanks. At this time, you can acknowledge the many contributions and sacrifices made by the organization's individuals and teams. Because these individuals and teams worked toward common goals with great determination, the hospital has a much brighter future. Here it is okay to use the word *closure*. The closure process should be done thoughtfully, and with dignity. During the turnaround phase, many difficult decisions were made. Many of these decisions were not made through a consensus decision-making or majority-rule process. Some people may say, great job! Others may have different opinions. Some people may have had their confidence shaken or feelings hurt. Others may be stronger for the experience. These two extremes in mind-set, and all those in between, are natural in a turnaround. Orchestrating the right closure process can start the healing and recovery process. Whether you believe a healing and recovery process is in order or not is probably irrelevant. Do it anyway. Never miss an opportunity to reach out and say thank you!

PIVOTING TO THE FUTURE

The second purpose of a celebration is to pivot from the turn-around era to the post-turnaround era. The post-turnaround era is where the groundwork for the future is framed and articulated. Although conventional wisdom seems to indicate the importance of allowing people to take some time to breathe and reflect on what has been accomplished, too much time in the pivot process can slow progress. The timing of this is a judgment call. You need to be able to gauge the hospital team's emotional state of mind in the consideration process. Seek out the advice of others as you contemplate this decision.

As you construct a framework for the future, consider these basic building blocks essential to any well-run organization:

- Vision
- Culture
- Values
- Annual operating plans
- Performance measurement systems
- Performance-based personnel evaluation systems

Vision

Create a bold and inspiring shared vision for the organization. Describe where you want your organization to be in five years—one of the best hospitals in the country, a regional leader in specific clinical services, recognized as physician-friendly hospital, or recognized employer of choice. Whatever vision you choose, talk about it often and with confidence. Nurture a passion for the vision within the team. Create measurable milestones in the journey towards the vision. Make the vision simple to understand and simple to remember.

Culture

Culture describes how your organization works. Create a culture of excellence. Strive for excellence in everything you do and all that every employee does within the organization. Excellence should not be an exclusive term. Yes, it should apply to quality, clinical outcomes, and patient experiences, but it should apply with equal zeal to the employee work environment, financial performance, and operational efficiency. Develop an environment that turns *average* into a four-letter word.

Values

A values statement is a set of shared beliefs promoted through the words or behavior of the people within a group or organization. Values speak to the conduct and behavior of individuals and organizations. Most hospitals have a values statement, and for organizations evolving out of a financial turnaround, values will continue to be important post-turnaround. One of the most frequent values appearing in a statement is teamwork. This is a good step, but for teamwork to be most effective, mutual accountability is required. Mutual accountability means that each individual on the team has an obligation to produce the desired results, and each member on the team has an obligation to hold others accountable for their performance as well. Mutual accountability can be difficult to pull off. Sometimes an individual may have to move outside his comfort level to hold others accountable for performance. But it should be encouraged and practiced. Results improve when teamwork improves.

Annual Operating Plan

Develop and implement an annual operating plan. The operating plan should contain the hospital's top 100 SMART (specific, measurable, assignable, realistic, and time-limited) objectives. The objectives should originate from the strategies and goals found in the organization's strategic plan. An operating plan is a tool for mutual accountability and consensus building in the post-turnaround era. Gather great input from top leadership to rank-and-file employees when developing the document. Once it is completed, share it with all stakeholders regularly.

Performance Management System

Develop a performance management system. Make sure it is process- and outcome-oriented. Within the management system, develop key performance indicators, balanced scorecards, dashboards, and a reporting system. Do not limit management and measurement systems to the senior executives. These tools should be in every department and all nursing units. Progress and barriers to success in achieving the measurements should be routinely communicated. The measurement systems should at a minimum cover the four areas of quality, finance, efficiency, and effectiveness.

Performance-Based Personnel Evaluation System

Develop a performance-based personnel evaluation system. Ensure the content of the evaluation system is reflective of the mission, vision, values, and annual operating plan of the organization. The system should encourage growth and development and mirror the desired objectives to be accomplished in the annual operating plan. Make sure all employees are evaluated, at least annually, from the CEO down to rank-and-file employees.

If a leader has these basic building blocks in her toolkit, she will have a great start to the post-turnaround era and future success.

A LAST WORD OF ADVICE

Develop an outcome-oriented leadership philosophy, and recognize your organization's most valuable asset is its people. Just as numbers will determine the long-term course of an organization, so will relationships. The post-turnaround era is a time to be mindful of both.

Financial Turnaround Cases

You HAVE NOW READ best practice approaches for identifying early warning signs of financial distress; making distinctions between symptoms and causes of financial distress; conducting diagnostic tests of the hospital operating environment, including the use of problem-solving drill-down techniques; developing communication plans with stakeholders; developing action plans in preparation for a turnaround; and implementing methods to ensure the most effective return on investment of time and resources. You have also read each chapter's Critical Success Factors (CSFs) to reinforce the learning process.

The following section presents a set of cases to challenge your thought process and put your newfound knowledge into action. These cases are constructed in a cross-functional manner that pulls you in multiple directions simultaneously. This tension creates discomfort because decisions are required quickly. This discomfort simulates the challenges in real-world turnarounds.

These cases can also be used in a group to spark the thought process—for example, with your executive team. The intent is not to labor over the case but rather to quickly apply and share what you have learned.

CASE 1: A PRIVATE, SECULAR HEALTHCARE SYSTEM

Three years ago Memorial Healthcare System, a private, secular system, wanted to significantly enhance its hospital–physician alignment strategy and become more competitive in the regional market as a provider of healthcare services. To accelerate this strategy, the two-hospital system executed a bold plan of purchasing as many physician practices as possible and hiring many physician specialists from the region and across the country. The acquisition and hiring blitz served two purposes. First, it was a defensive move to ensure the system's current market share and market position were not diminished through loss of providers. And second, it positioned the organization as a future player in the emerging population health management market by moving its providers to geographical areas historically dominated by its competitors.

Memorial wanted to provide excellent clinical services to as many patients and covered lives as possible and, in the process, constrain the flow of patients to its competitors. The system acquired primary care practices and hired specialists, including cardiologists, intensivists, surgeons, oncologists, and obstetrics/gynecologists. The system's excess cash levels funded these acquisitions and were invested in upgrading existing facilities and adding new ones. The majority of the physicians in the practice acquisitions and new hires preferred an employer–employee arrangement instead of private practice. It was fair to say a significant portion of the medical staff was economically tied to the healthcare system.

Three years after feverishly executing the new hospital–physician alignment strategy, the healthcare system was incredibly successful in adding new physicians, new patients, and new covered lives. Volume was up, and the number of covered lives increased.

But executing this massive hospital–physician alignment strategy at such a feverish pace had unintended consequences. The healthcare system experienced an increasing financial loss in its operating margin for the first time in ten years. This was something new to the current leadership. The first loss on the operating margin was 3 percent and occurred in the second year of deploying the strategy. The third year saw a 4 percent loss. The projected operating loss for the upcoming year is 6 percent. The industry average was a 3 percent loss on the operating margin. Factors contributing to the losses are multivariant. The once cash-rich healthcare system is no longer. The organization has set a modest goal of meeting the industry average for days cash on hand.

Consecutive annual financial losses are unacceptable, especially at the magnitude projected for the upcoming year. The urgency of the situation is compounded by the organization's decline in cash position.

Questions to Consider

1. Other than the operating margin, what metrics can be used to measure the financial health of the organization?
2. What steps would you take to address this situation? What would you do first?
3. What went right for the organization in this situation?
4. What went wrong for the organization in this situation? How do you know this?
5. Identify leadership shortfalls in this situation, if any.
6. What are some of the pitfalls and potential leadership tipping points in this situation?
7. Construct a burning platform for this situation. What would the central message be?

CASE 2: A PUBLIC HOSPITAL

Johnson County Medical Center (JCMC) is a publicly owned 500-bed hospital serving an indigent population in a large metropolitan area. JCMC has a very good reputation for providing access to the underserved populations in the community. Unfortunately, it also has the image of being the hospital of last resort. The depth and breadth of its services are well known, from its high-end tertiary services, such as neurosurgery and cardiovascular surgery, to the geographically dispersed primary care services in the clinics. A 20-member board of directors oversees the day-to-day operations and fiscal resources of JCMC. The board members are appointed by the county commission for staggered three-year terms. The majority of the medical staff is provided by the local medical school, a relationship that dates back 30 to 40 years. The hospital also directly employs a number of physicians unrelated to the medical school. Most employees are represented by two major unions. Employee morale is a concern because of the constant discussions around the financial viability of the organization, given its challenges. Because of these challenges, a rash of recent rumors about impending layoffs have taken root. These rumors have obviously caused a level of uncertainty throughout the environment.

Approximately 60 percent of the hospital's total patient population are Medicaid recipients and the uninsured. Medicare and commercial insurance patients account for only 15 percent and 10 percent, respectively. The rest of the hospital's funding is in grants from local, state, and federal agencies. Despite JCMC's best efforts, most of its patients used the emergency department as their first option for receiving primary care treatment. Remarkably, in an annual ranking of patient satisfaction in metropolitan hospitals, JCMC has been positioned in the middle of the pack and sometimes near the top of the list in certain categories.

Over the years, JCMC has struggled financially for many reasons: lack of insured patients, operational inefficiencies, patient throughput challenges, quality-of-care concerns, and the episodic nature of care to most of the population it serves. The county government has subsidized JCMC for decades. Over the past ten years, the county's subsidy to JCMC has been rising at a rate well beyond the consumer price index and well beyond the rise in expenses at other local hospitals. The county subsidy is 20 percent of JCMC's total annual operating budget. More concerning to the county commission, which decides how much to allocate to JCMC each year, is how much of the county's budget JCMC is increasingly taking. Commissioners are worried about what impact these JCMC increases will have on the provision of other county services. Even with the 20 percent subsidy, JCMC has had 4 to 5 percent operating losses for the past three years. These losses have been covered by specially appropriated state funds in the form of grants. However, the state and county governments have signaled that they are no longer willing to provide these levels of subsidies to JCMC. The hospital needs to overhaul itself and improve its performance. The county commission has asked for a turnaround plan with execution strategies.

Questions to Consider

1. How will you address the county commissioners' concerns? Include the political and image implications of the government's request.
2. With whom will you consult and speak first as you respond to the request for a turnaround plan?
3. What will the turnaround plan look like? Is it possible to develop a plan that makes JCMC financially viable in the minds of the commissioners and the public?
4. How will you engage the board of directors in the process? What role should the board play in this turnaround effort?

5. Articulate a burning platform in light of the fact that the organization has historically been losing money on its operations.
6. How will you address the rumors running rampant among employees?

CASE 3: AN ACADEMIC MEDICAL CENTER

University Hospital (UH) is a 400-bed institution located in a major metropolitan area. It is part of a prestigious private academic medical center that includes a nationally recognized medical school and research foundation that has received millions in grants from the National Institutes of Health (NIH). Formerly owned by the university, the hospital is now a private, freestanding institution. Because of the major financial liabilities that come with running a hospital in today's healthcare market, the university sought to limit its liabilities and sold majority ownership to a 501(c)3 not-for-profit organization. The university retained a 20 percent ownership stake in the institution. The hospital has a 25-member board of directors, five of whom are appointed by the university's board of directors and four of whom are appointed by the school of medicine, as stipulated by the sale agreement.

The hospital's market share is consistent with its size and scope of services. UH's market share has not changed much in the five years since the sale, and there has been significant downward pressure on hospital costs from payers and the public no longer wishing to pay a premium price for services found at comparable institutions.

Three years ago, UH started losing money on its operations. The losses have grown in each of the past three successive years. Revenues are flat because of tightening reimbursement. Costs are still high because the hospital is part of an academic enterprise with major teaching responsibilities. The hospital's operating losses have been offset by its interest income from endowment funds and philanthropic contributions. However, the use of these funds has drawn the attention of several influential board members who are also major benefactors of the hospital. These board members believe the earned interest income should be used for direct investments in clinical programs and facilities, not to offset operating losses.

A recent metro market study showed the gap has narrowed significantly in the public's perception of quality of care at UH and other competing hospitals. For pricing and cost reasons, insurers and patients are indicating a willingness to look at other institutions beyond UH. If UH starts to lose market share, its operating losses would increase even more. Of the more than 20 hospitals located in the UH metropolitan area, UH has the highest cost-per-discharge of any institution. The concern among the UH leadership is that UH's cost structure is out of line with its competitors, and this should be addressed. Other members of the board see the situation differently. A number of these board members are also faculty at the medical school. They have taken the position that UH and the academic medical center provide a unique service to the community in the form of cutting-edge medicine and state-of-the-art research. These unique contributions to the community should be recognized and factored into the value and cost equations. Further, no other facility like it exists in the region. These board members argued that no decision should be made that will damage the clinical reputation of the medical center.

Questions to Consider

1. Identify the key stakeholders in this situation.
2. Identify the differences between the stakeholders and stakeholder groups.
3. How would you approach a discussion with each stakeholder or stakeholder group?
4. Identify the political pain points for key stakeholders.
5. How would you devise a plan to get the various stakeholders on the same page?
6. Identify any symptoms and causes that may be contributing to UH's financial downturn.
7. Can an effective turnaround plan be developed for UH? If so, how would it be structured? Who would be the major players?

CASE 4: A RELIGIOUS HOSPITAL

St. Mary's Hospital is a 190-bed facility that has been serving its community for the past 110 years. Owned and operated by a national multihospital system corporation, St. Mary's has been faithfully pursuing its mission to serve underserved populations. Recognized for its dedication to this singular mission, the religious institution has been nationally recognized for its development of community outreach and preventive medicine programs in numerous underserved communities. Some of its most noted programs include hypertension clinics, chronic disease management of diabetes, maternal care for high-risk pregnancies, and prostate and breast cancer screening. St. Mary's was recently recognized as the Corporate Citizen of the Year by the state chamber of commerce. Despite all of these accolades, St. Mary's continues to struggle financially. The institution has struggled to balance its mission with its margin. It has a challenging payer mix that includes a large number of Medicaid patients and the uninsured. The hospital has not generated a positive operating margin in six years, and the losses are into millions of dollars.

During this time, the hospital's parent corporation has been subsidizing the losses. Even with the support of a national healthcare system behind it, the hospital has recently suffered another downgrade of its bonds—this time, to non-investment-grade status. The major concern of the bond market is the continuing decline of the facility's financial health and its perceived inability to attract more insured patients because of its location in a low-income neighborhood. At present, the hospital has single-digit days cash on hand. Meeting the biweekly payroll has been a challenge for years. To smooth over some of these financial problems, the corporate office has been providing temporary loans and bridge loans. Repayment of these loans is still pending, well beyond the original due dates.

The hospital's latest communication from the corporate office is to prepare a sound financial turnaround plan for the institution or prepare the organization for sale or closure. The hospital leadership team has decided to put a turnaround plan in place. However, they have attempted this before with limited success.

Word of the corporate office's decision has filtered back to the employees at the institution. Many are concerned about their job security. Some employees are signaling that looking for an opportunity in a more stable organization in the community would be a sound idea. The president of the medical staff has requested a meeting with administration to discuss the rumors. A core group of physicians have been loyal to the institution, but they are now questioning whether this is time to start redirecting their admissions to more stable competing hospitals. The local hospital board has limited power and authority. Many major decisions rest with the parent board of directors, but the local leadership has control of the cost structure and clinical programs administration. The board chair and hospital CEO have been in constant communications about the issues and situation. They both agree a special board meeting should be called to discuss the status of the hospital and any go-forward plans.

Questions to Consider

1. How should the hospital CEO prepare for this meeting?
2. What should be the first step in the turnaround process?
3. Who are the major stakeholders in this situation?
4. What is required to develop a sound financial turnaround plan?
5. Who should be involved in the development of this plan?
6. How would you deal with the employees' and medical staff's apprehensions about organizational instability?
7. St. Mary's tried a turnaround plan previously and was unsuccessful. How will you ensure success this time around?

CASE 5: A SUBURBAN HOSPITAL

Suburban Hospital is a 225-bed for-profit institution purchased by a national multihospital system from a religious institution about nine months ago. The hospital is located in a middle-class community where the majority of the population has insurance, but the level of the uninsured is continuing to rise. Along with the rise in the uninsured is the rise in uncompensated care. Prior to the for-profit corporation's purchase, the religious institution had consistently struggled with financial losses. Investments in clinical programs and facilities had nearly come to a halt because of the lack of capital and a declining market for the institution's debt. Physicians and patients frequently complained that the institution lagged behind community standards in the quality of its facilities.

Based on the institution's inability to compete in quality of facilities, the public started drawing conclusions that the quality of care was substandard as well. This was not true, and the hospital's quality could be proven in clinical outcome comparison. However, this was the public perception. Volume was steadily declining and had dropped by 15 percent over the past several years. The drop in volume could be directly connected to the decline in physician loyalty to the institution. Physicians were increasingly admitting their patients to competitors.

When the religious institution sold the hospital to the for-profit corporation, it had been losing money on its operations for the previous five years. The most recent annual loss was 6 percent on the operating margin.

With the change in ownership came new leadership for the hospital and a directive to develop a written turnaround plan within the next 45 days to have the hospital operating in the black within six months.

Questions to Consider

1. Where would you start?
2. Can you identify the key stakeholders? Specifically, within each stakeholder group, with whom would you speak?
3. Can you identify quick fixes versus long-term fixes for improvement?
4. How would you map out your plan? At the end of 45 days, what would your plan look like?

CASE 6: MEDICAL STAFF: A STAKEHOLDER MANAGEMENT AND COMMUNICATIONS PLAN

Southern Medical Center (Southern) has a well-established reputation in the local community as a friendly place. Patient satisfaction and employee satisfaction scores are some of the highest in the region. The hospital is most noted for being a physician-friendly institution. In a recent physician satisfaction survey, Southern was rated highest in responsiveness to physician needs. Executive leadership has concluded that these numbers offer a strategic advantage in the highly competitive local market. Hospital leadership has relied on these relationships to drive patient volume and covered lives to the facility for years. Although hospital leadership had viewed these relationships as a market leverage point, times are changing. Most decisions involve good relationships, but the crucial leverage point has turned out to be economics.

Because of a declining revenue base and escalating operating costs, Southern has been losing money for the past two years. During a deep-dive discussion last week, the executive team concluded that the financial decline has three major contributors: operational inefficiencies, a loss in market share to competitors, and expensive loss-leader clinical programs. The operational inefficiencies include a higher-than-average patient length of stay and slow turnaround time for key services, which is driving labor costs to be among the highest in the community. The loss in market share came at the hands of a successful competitor, Eastern Hospital. Four years ago, Eastern initiated a major building program on its main campus. It established a leadership role in several clinical services it was previously struggling in by recruiting marquee physicians from competitors, mainly Southern. Eastern has acquired several large, high-profile physician practices and relocated them within a mile of Southern. Today, Eastern is the dominant hospital in the service area, mostly at the expense of Southern. Many of the physicians pushing the competitive edge at Eastern are former Southern loyalists. After conducting a profit and loss analysis of each clinical service line, the leadership was able to identify clinical programs generating financial losses. Some of these clinical programs were major loss leaders. They were high-volume programs, but every admission and outpatient visit incurred incremental losses. To complicate the situation, several of these programs were tied to major admitting physician groups and hospital loyalists. How the issues surrounding the loss-leader program are handled could affect relationships with the affected physicians and the medical staff.

To date, the executive leadership team has resisted the prospect of implementing a major turnaround plan for fear of alienating the medical staff and influential physicians. However, last week in consultation with the board of directors, the executive team moved forward with a comprehensive turnaround plan that will include a review of operational efficiencies, labor costs, supply costs, managed care contracts, and loss-leader clinical programs. As expected, there will be many moving parts to this turnaround. In this case, focus on how you would deal with the medical staff.

Questions to Consider

1. How would you manage a key stakeholder in the hospital—the medical staff?
2. If you were limited to five talking points with the medical staff about the turnaround, what would they be?
3. Who would you engage in the turnaround discussions and medical staff discussions?
4. How would you handle push back from the medical staff on the turnaround plan?
5. How would the discussions and decisions regarding the continuation or elimination of loss-leader clinical programs be handled?

CASE 7: THE EMPLOYEES: A STAKEHOLDER MANAGEMENT AND COMMUNICATIONS PLAN

Southwestern Medical Center is a 350-bed hospital with a workforce of 1,400 employees. It has an annual operating budget of $220 million but has lost money on its operations for years. It has resisted the prospect of employee staff reductions because this was generally viewed as not consistent with the organization's goal of remaining an employer of choice. However, the hospital's finances were declining precipitously 11 months ago, and it laid off 40 full-time equivalent (FTE) employees in a one-month period. At the time, it was thought the layoffs would stem the losses, which were approaching 3.5 percent for a second year in a row. The tactic did not eliminate the losses, but it did slow them down.

The prospects for a financial recovery do not look promising unless a comprehensive plan can be developed to address many of Southwestern's issues related to performance. These issues are broad and sweeping and include labor and non-labor areas. In collaborations with the board of directors and medical staff, leadership concluded that a turnaround plan had to be developed and implemented within 60 days. The potential staff reductions in the turnaround plan will exceed those made 11 months ago. Rumors about more staff reductions are swirling throughout the hospital.

Questions to Consider

1. As part of a comprehensive turnaround plan, develop an outline of a stakeholder management and communications plan for employees.

2. In the communications plan, how will you explain the need to implement a second staff reduction in such a short span of time?
3. As you develop the plan, identify some of the major pitfalls and issues that will be a challenge along the way.

CASE 8: DEFINING THE BOARD'S ROLE IN A FINANCIAL TURNAROUND

Community Medical Center (CMC) is a 250-bed hospital with several ambulatory care centers and owned physician practices. It is one of ten hospitals in the community, but only one of four for tertiary services. CMC's finances have been a concern for years. Last year, a lengthy newspaper article was written on the financial challenges at the medical center. The article places some of the blame on an ineffective board of directors—some of whom have extensive tenure but lack obvious skill sets—among many other reasons. You have been recruited to lead a turnaround at the institution. The board has called a special session to meet with you. They want you to make a presentation on your turnaround plan.

You will have one hour for the presentation, and you should be prepared to field questions along the way. The board is most interested in how you see their role in the turnaround. They take great pride in being a hands-on group when it comes to the day-to-day operations of the hospital. They have signaled they expect to be very involved in this turnaround process.

Questions to Consider

1. Prepare an outline of your turnaround plan presentation to the board. What will you include?
2. Define the board's role and how you see the working relationship moving forward.

References

American Hospital Association (AHA). 2013. "Trendwatch Chart-book." Accessed January 28, 2013. www.aha.org/research/reports/tw/chartbook/index.shtml.

Gladwell, M. 2002. *The Tipping Point: How Little Things Can Make a Big Difference.* Boston: Back Bay Books.

Health Care Advisory Board. 2000. *Radical Turnarounds: Key Lessons from Hospital and Health System Case Studies.* Accessed January 25, 2013. www.advisory.com/Research/Health-Care-Advisory-Board/Studies/2000/Radical-Turnarounds.

Rindler, M. 2002. *Essential Guide to Managing Consultants.* Chicago: Health Administration Press.

Safabi, K. 2007. "Revenue and Productivity Are Keys to Profitability." *Healthcare Financial Management* December 1, 5–6.

Index

Academic medical centers (AMCs),
107–11, 119
case study, 133–34
Accountability, 97–98
of chief executive officers (CEOs),
17–21
identification of lapses in, 20, 21
as motivation for financial turnarounds, 32–33, 42–43
mutual, 123, 124
organizational culture of, 12
of public hospitals, 114
Accounts payable, 4, 75
Accounts receivable, 75
Acid test, of financial performance,
2, 3–4
Acquisitions, as financial distress
cause, 10, 11
Action plans, targeted, 56, 58, 59
Administrative expenses, data availability about, 60
Admissions
increase in, as revenue strategy,
62, 63
trends in, as financial performance
indicator, 3, 4
Asset-based lending, 62
Assets, noncore, divestiture of, 62,
81, 84

Audit tools, 72–73
Average days in accounts receivable, 3
Average length of stay (ALOS), 60

Balanced scorecards, 71, 77, 124
Balance sheets, 11, 65, 71, 81
Benchmarking data and tools, 58,
59, 71, 78, 91
in hotwiring approach, 79–80
sources and availability of, 2–3,
59–60
Best practices, 74
data sources for, 59–60
Billing cycle, 68
Billing systems, improvement of, 63
Board of directors
communication with, 27, 45–48,
143
concerns about financial turnarounds, 40–41, 47–48
questions about financial turnarounds, 45–48, 143
support for financial turnarounds,
85
Bond ratings, as financial performance indicators, 7
Bridge financing, 61
Budget management, with electronic
financial management systems, 75

Messages
altruistic, 42–43, 44
combined, 44
as communication process/plan
component, 24, 25–26, 28,
33–34, 35
concrete results, 43
self-preservation, 43–44
Middle managers
relationships with vendors, 91
roles and responsibilities, 87, 91,
92
Mission and mission statements
of academic medical centers,
109–10
altruistic, 42
bottom line and, 24
of for-profit hospitals, 117
as operating loss cause, 8
of public hospitals, 115
of religious hospitals, 111, 112
Mistakes
admission of, 17–20, 30
in communication process/plans,
29–30, 31–32, 35
strategic, as financial distress
cause, 10, 11
Mortality and morbidity indicators,
60

"No message, no mission," 112
Notes payable, converting to, 61
Nursing units, full-time equivalent
employees of, 87

Objectives
clinical outcome, 43

discussion in communication pro-
cess/plans, 32
financial, 43
operational, 43
responsibility for accomplishment
of, 20
SMART (specific, measurable,
assignable, realistic, and time-
limited), 123–24
Operating budgets, 79–80
Operating losses, causes of, 8–13
Operating margins, 3, 4, 6, 8, 9
Operating plans, annual, 123–24
Operating rooms, improved turnaround in, 63–64
Operational efficiency. See Efficiency
Organizational characteristics, affecting financial turnarounds, 107–19
of academic medical centers,
107–11, 119
of for-profit hospitals, 116–18
of public hospitals, 113–16
of religious hospitals, 111–13
Organizational culture
of accountability, 12
of excellence, 123
as financial distress cause, 8,
10–11, 12
Organizational structure, as financial
distress cause, 10–11
Overtime utilization reports, 79–80
Ownership status. See
Organizational characteristics

Patient care champions, 87
Patient discharges, from hospitals.
See Discharges

About the Author

Anthony K. (Tony) Jones is a veteran healthcare and hospital industry expert with substantial experience improving the performance of financially distressed hospitals. He holds a master's degree in health administration from St. Louis University and an undergraduate degree from Abilene Christian University. Jones started his career in the public hospital sector, serving two different systems in Michigan. This experience of consistently having limited resources and outsized demand for services brought his attention to the need to have hospitals operate at optimal efficiency to achieve their mission.

Assuming substantial senior management responsibilities early in his career helped accelerate his understanding of how hospitals operate strategically and down to the ground level, including the delivery of care at the patient bedside. Working with boards of directors, medical staffs, and senior management groups, Jones has assisted hospitals in distress across all sectors of the industry: public hospitals, faith-based institutions, multihospital systems, and academic medical centers. He was appointed administrator of a 300-bed, private, not-for-profit safety net hospital in southern New Jersey. Two years later, he was appointed chief operating officer of a private, not-for-profit, two-hospital system in northern New Jersey. Both organizations were in financial distress. He was able to transform both institutions significantly by improving their operational and financial performance. Later, he served as CEO of a 600-bed religious hospital and COO of a 500-bed for-profit hospital. All of these experiences had a powerful impact on his understanding of what it takes to be successful in financially transforming a hospital while maintaining high-quality care and improving employee morale.

Tony Jones is an industry consultant, speaker, and author in health and hospital management. He can be reached at (678) 920-0882.